The Secrets of Longevity

By

Dr Joseph Cheung

The author

Dr Cheung, OAM, was brought up in Hong Kong, the third son in a family of five. His father was an ENT professor at Sun Yat Sen University in Canton, China, and also a noted authority on the herbs of Hong Kong for which he wrote the classic textbook used to this day.

Joseph and his brothers, Nelson and Stanley, who were to become noted medical men like himself, studied hard and practised sports and he developed a lifelong love of exercise and belief in its benefits.

In the 1950s Dr Cheung went to Australia to study medicine and he graduated from the University of Sydney in 1960. Thereafter, followed stints at Hong Kong's Kwong Wah Hospital and in Toronto Canada at the university of Ottawa. There he studied pathology under Professor D Magner, the head of the Canadian Tumour Registry, and the Department of Pathology of the University of Ottawa. Joseph participated in research into renal transplants and ovarian cancer, and in publications on those topics.

After returning to Australia and settling into a medical clinic in Melbourne, Dr Cheung continued to practise what he preached by swimming and jogging daily. Over the years, he started to notice the therapeutic benefits of Oriental medical practices such as acupuncture and Tai Chi. He has since fervently promoted these aids to health to his patients, with excellent results, as published in his article in the *American Journal of Chinese Medicine* in 1985 and detailed in his first book, *Total Health and Fitness Revolution*, published in 2012.

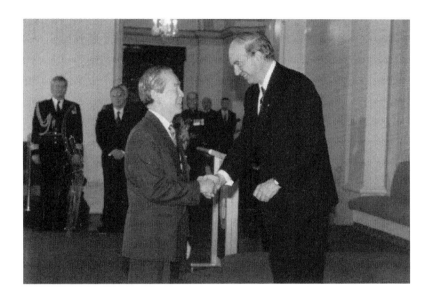

His proudest moment came in 1998 when he was awarded the Medal of the Order of Australia (OAM) on Australia Day, for his service to medicine and the community, in particular, to the Australian Chinese Medical Association.

Foreword

By **Dr Kin Liu**

Dr Joseph Cheung has been a dedicated General Medical Practitioner in Glenroy, Victoria since 1971 and then subsequently in Epping, Sydney from 2010 till his retirement in 2020. He has devoted all his life to community service and was awarded the Member of the Order of Australia in 1998.

I have had the honour of being his acquaintance and have been associated with him for over thirty odd years. He is a dedicated, kind and gentle General Practitioner and always willing to share his knowledge with his patients and colleagues. The combination of his skills in Eastern and Western medicine and his compassion has helped him to be a highly successful medical doctor.

Joseph was also a dedicated member of the Victorian Chinese Medical Association and was elected as its president in 1994. His previous acclaimed book, entitled *Total Health and Fitness Revolution* or 青春健康美新论 (Chinese), was a great success and is well worth reading.

After his recent retirement from medical practice, at the ripe age of 87, he has decided to write this book Unlocking the Secrets of Longevity in which he shares his lifelong "East- West anti-aging" knowledge with his readers.

Joseph's new book starts with a tour of the World's Centenarian Blue Zones followed by "Reflections" from the Blue Zones and then finishes with the challenges and prevention of Longevity, including the "Hi-tech Dragon".

He shares his daily routine and secret advice with his readers, including

1. Regular and stretching exercises
2. Dietary and calorie measurements
3. Relaxation and sleep patterns
4. Usage of medical supplements

This book will benefit all age groups

for many years to come. Dr Kin Liu
MBBS {Melb}, FRACR
Radiologist
Founder of Diagnostic Imaging Group, Melbourne

Table of Contents

Important vegetables and their properties . 189

Melons, sprouts, fungi and more...................... 196

Introduction: Unlocking the Secrets of Longevity

After sixty years serving society as a medical doctor and medical acupuncturist in various countries over three continents, I got the crazy idea in my head that I should keep on working, day in and day out, diagnosing and treating illnesses in a wide variety of patients of many ethnic origins; I should also continue chatting with all sorts of people: not just patients, but also learned colleagues, specialists, nursing staff, managers and the seemingly never-ending parade of those talkative representatives from pharmaceutical companies. It has all been very congenial and pleasant working as a team in this way; an enjoyable and motivating phase of my medical career.

Hardly anyone ever asked me when I would retire, or if, in fact, I had any intention of retiring at all. Occasionally an old patient might ask my age, which I took as a kind of hint that maybe I should be thinking of retirement. "Not to worry," I'd tell them. "I am still fit and healthy, and have no problem managing my heavy patient load yet." Sometimes, I'd crack a joke about aiming to be the oldest GP in Australia. I'd say I would like to keep consulting "until I drop". "That's terrific, doc, we like to stick to the one doctor," some would say. "My family are happy to see you forever." Such expressions of appreciation, right from the heart of one's loyal patients, were not uncommon in general practice in Australia in the old days, but I fear they will be getting rarer and rarer in future because of diminishing face-to-face contact and shrinking consultation times. Nevertheless, moments like those are surely one of the motivations for GPs to keep working and trying their best to help their patients.

"You don't need to retire if you reckon you can still work," said my brother Stanley. He's a few years younger than me but retired many years ago because of tremendous work pressure from working as one of the top neurosurgeons in Hong Kong. He declares that "General practice is easy, no worries at night. And do you know Dr Blackburn Sr, the vice chancellor of Sydney University was still looking after patients at the age of ninety-something?'

However, enter the coronavirus, everything started to change, and had to change – and so has my medical life.

For anyone who has never gone through the stages of retirement before, this decision to abruptly cease your rather hectic daily routine of an early morning swim, rushing through breakfast and driving to the clinic in the morning to take care of all sorts of patients before going through the peak hour traffic to get back home, with more to do at home – cooking, washing up and never ending paperwork – feels like a major event, not unlike a mini-bomb exploding nearby. For moments after, your mind has gone blank and you have to scratch your brain to re-ignite the fire and do a great deal of soul-searching and planning in regard to what to do next.

I have always been interested in keeping fit and practising regular exercise so that I can withstand the trauma and strain common to general medical practice. Since my early teens, I have built up knowledge in this area from swimming coaches, talks, research and lots of personal experience with regular training and competitive swimming in Hong Kong. And then, after starting a family and settling down to work in general practice, I developed a daily jogging routine. I even did a one-off marathon in Melbourne. To cap off all these efforts and to attempt to influence many of my patients to follow a healthy and active life, I wrote my first book *Total Health and Fitness Revolution*, which initially sold mainly to my clinical patients but is now available from Amazon in print and as an e-book. Many of my readers have told me how much they appreciate my teaching and advice on health matters and fitness training. Some have bought extra copies as gifts for their friends and relatives so that they too can learn how to be fitter and healthier.

When a person has advanced far enough in their journey of life, at some stage they start to realize that life is not the infinitive oasis it seemed to be when they were in their teens. Life itself, like everything else around us, is a finite form of all living matter – it will wear out, it will degenerate, it will disintegrate into a void, an emptiness in the end. The infinite oasis will prove to be a mirage which eventually disappears. Even the great Chinese scholar and philosopher Confucius admitted to his disciples, birth and death – the two greatest events of life – were baffling and incomprehensible to him.

There is a most famous Chinese poem of exceptional length, *The Song of Anguished Love* by the famed poet Bai Ger Yee which was written during the great Tong Dynasty. In it, the poet lavishes his powerful poetic gifts on recording and describing the beautiful and intimate love between the emperor and his enchanting and alluring concubine. She died tragically, being executed in front of the emperor by the revolting army. So great was his grief that he cried tears filled with blood. The last two verses are particularly moving. They describe the emperor's enduring tender heart-broken love as an infinitively sweet but sad dream lasting forever:

> The vast sky and the solid land may have a limit sometimes; but the broken love and enduring sorrow will flow on and on forever to eternity.

It seems that only poets and artists possess the intuition that emotion, feeling, and tender love can infuse the universe forever as something infinite.

From my long-held interest in exercise and fitness, I have gained an intuition of a different kind, hinting to me that this could be the first step into the tunnel to longevity. And indeed, as soon as my son David had picked up the latest copy of a book on longevity by Professor D. Sinclair and posted to me, followed not long after with another thick volume by Professor L. Fontana, I knew immediately that I had got a lot of ammunition to start working on this fascinating biological enigma of life and death, longevity, ageing, chronic medical illness, and the deep-down subcellular metabolism. They all intertwine to be part and parcel of the phenomenon we call lifespan.

This knowledge is something new to me and other GPs and specialists trained traditionally in medical schools. It has enabled us to find out how a single fertilised egg can swiftly develop into a complex embryo and then a fully formed foetus possessing limbs, a brain and internal organs, as if a pre-set program has been turned on by someone. We now also know why a person slowly 'wears out', ages, and suffers illnesses such as cancer. The teaching of medical students in Australia, when I was studying, post-WWII, was pretty stereotypically textbook style – attending lectures, reading books, doing simple basic lab work on superficial procedures and experiments occasionally. There were very few inspirational lectures and talks by visiting eminent researchers and scientists. There was also a huge knowledge deficit in medical teaching and university lab research, as if medical students needed only know how to make clinical diagnoses and what medications to use to treat diseases, and then off these new doctors went into the world to take care of patients and build up their wealth. There is a wise saying in a passage I have read that "people spend too much time making money and not enough time caring about their health, so they end up in retirement rich in wealth so they are unable to spend it all, but poor in health too late to repair" – what an honest reminder! And so true to the bone too!

Of the many books on the topic of longevity that I have read, Professor D. Sinclair's *Lifespan* has been one of the few that really opened my eyes to the world of life and death, the world of lab animal experiments, the world of scientific logic and hard work, and the world of the miracle that exists in our every cell, which conducts numerous biochemical reactions day in and day out, at nano scale, controlled by our genes, DNA and feed-back mechanisms, in a perfectly orderly fashion. Sometimes these processes are mind boggling, and often they are even beyond our imagination, but, above all, they are absolutely exciting.

Inspired by this, I made an in-depth study of the work of many demographers (specialists in population statistics). Having combined that study with a consideration of the opinions and explanations of other authors, scientists, and investigative journalists, finally the ageing process does not appear to be such an elusive phenomenon. So, I have made up my mind to present, in a simplified form, the phenomenon of longevity by writing this book with the following purposes:

Firstly, to inform general readers interested in the hitherto mysterious phenomenon of ageing just how its cryptic nature has been slowly revealed.

Secondly, to inspire my readers to adopt a healthy lifestyle which includes first and foremost a regular exercise routine on top of sensible diet to achieve a healthier, more energetic and happier existence and a longer lifespan. Such practices can be expected to simultaneously help protect us from dreaded cancers and chronic diseases that could only bring pain, suffering and misery. In the same breath, however, I must remind the readers that this strategy cannot be one hundred per cent foolproof as longevity also involves other factors such as heredity, environment and community influences, which must also be taken into consideration. While there are doubtless still exciting discoveries yet to be made, by practising the advice contained in this book, you should be able to push back ageing much more effectively than uninformed and chronic "couch potatoes" will be able to do. You are bound to wind up happier than you would be otherwise, due to being spared many chronic painful disabilities and illnesses. You will, in fact, ensure that you have the best chance of avoiding all disease completely.

Dr Joseph Cheung

Acknowledgements

The book is a tribute to my late father who has dedicated his whole life to the advancement of Chinese medicinal herbalism in Hong Kong.

This book in many ways is very different from my first one, which focuses mainly on health, fitness and the prevention of the various medical diseases I had become extremely familiar with during my forty years of general medical practice. The current volume relies heavily on the latest scientific information, research findings and lab experiments done globally.

I am also fortunate to receive never-ending support and encouragement from my brother Stanley, one of the most brilliant and beloved neurosurgeons in Hong Kong, who retired from his hectic neurosurgical practice years ago, and the same from my two intelligent and sensible children, my son David and my daughter Deborah, who are both hardworking doctors. Sincere thanks also go to many of my former colleagues and regular meet-groups both in Victoria and Sydney who keep me on the go, and in particular a special personal Big Thankyou to Dr Kin Liu, the hard-working founder and head of the powerful Diagnostic Imaging Group of Melbourne, for his generous foreword, to say nothing of our thirty years of personal and professional friendship.

I would also like to thank my editor Jan Scherpenhuizen for his never-ending professional guidance and great assistance.

Finally I would like to express my appreciation to all the scientists and researchers whose persistent efforts and dedication are helping to de-mystifying this inscrutable disease – ageing – to the benefit of us all. Their names appear as authors of their reference books in this work. I have learnt so much from their work, which has impressed upon me, more than ever, the validity of the Chinese saying 'knowledge knows no boundaries'.

Dr Joseph Cheung

Chapter One: In Search of a Longer Lifespan during the Covid-19 Pandemic

For those of us living with all the privileges of the developed world, everything must have seemed pretty rosy until the bombshell exploded at the end of 2019. A new coronavirus had entered our lives. Structurally, it is thought to be quite similar to the SARS virus that initiated an epidemic in Hong Kong and southern China nearly ten years ago, and to the Ebola virus in Africa. At the time of writing, an expert team of scientific investigators organised by the World Health Organisation (WHO), after a month's investigation in January-February 2021, has made it clear that the point of origin of the disease cannot be definitively identified. However, it seems most likely that the new disease started its massive spread from a wet market in Wu Han, the capital of Hu Bei province in China. As it was begun during the ten days' festive holiday of Chinese New Year, which is enjoyed by most Chinese, tens of thousands of holiday makers, visitors and tourists all mixed together. This led to them unknowingly spreading the virus, which raged like a bushfire through most parts of China and eventually every country in the world.

The WHO had no option but to declare the situation a pandemic as the virus continued its relentless march and reached one hundred and sixty-eight or more nations. The disease was officially named COVID-19. Up to 15 August 2020, the world had reported over twenty-three million people infected and over eight hundred thousand deaths, mostly of people over sixty, many of whom died of pneumonia and lung complications while being treated on respirators in ICUs. Hospitals and medical centres all over the world suddenly found themselves facing crises because they were not equipped to handle the daily rising flood of sick patients infected with the virus. They rapidly ran out of beds for these patients, and make-shift hospitals had to be set up in large buildings like indoor football stadiums and public halls.

China, the origin of the pandemic, with its vast population and densely packed cities, would normally have been expected to be among the worst hit nations when it came to the death rate. Surprisingly, however, it happened to be the first one to get the infection under control due to a series of border lockdowns and strict quarantines, in addition to the speedy construction of huge new hospitals for patients with more complications, particularly with respiratory functions. On the other hand, more advanced health care nations like the US, UK and some EU countries have been left far behind in the overall strategy on infection control, anti-viral PPI (personal protection items or equipment) and in the effectiveness of lockdown of COVID-19 hot spots, so much so that the USA, the world's number one power, recorded the highest number of positive cases in 2020 and a shocking number of deaths. Claims of "fake news" do not deserve to be taken seriously, for all the mileage Donald Trump attempted to make of it, and by the end of his presidency on 20 January 2021 well over four hundred thousand Americans had lost their lives to the disease. Despite the massive immunisation programme rolled out, the death rate continues to remain high at this time. The open bickering between President Trump and many state governors over COVID-19, as well as Trump's insensitivity to the BLM movement, seemed to pour oil on the fire, resulting in mass demonstrations and civil unrest, night after night, and the inevitable chaotic looting and destruction of public properties. What a mess! What followed, including the US election drama and the insurrection of Trump's followers ending up in deadly rioting where five people died and a number of federal buildings were ransacked at the Capitol on 6 Jan 2021, is now a matter of history.

So, this is the COVID-19 pandemic, a once-in-a-century catastrophe, and the year 2020 will be the year that many wish had never arrived, and yet few will forget the huge loss of lives, astronomical unemployment rates and long-lasting economic horror inflicted on the world.

That was the setting in which I came to reassess my crazy idea of practising medicine until I drop. The coronavirus was crazier than I could ever be. The global lockdowns upset everyone's lives, greatly restricting our freedom to move around, to visit and socialise with friends and relatives, to enjoy ourselves in a restaurant. We couldn't even go shopping when we wanted to, or go wherever we wanted to. My dream of looking forward to being one of the longest serving GPs in Australia was just another of the many casualties of the pandemic. The reason why is fairly obvious: being over eighty, I am well and truly in the highest risk category. Working as a doctor I have a high chance of catching the coronavirus from an asymptomatic but infected patient and dying from respiratory failure or cardiac complications.

Of course, medical consultation under the pandemic atmosphere has completely changed, maybe forever, along with shopping and dining, to a new form. Now the norm is on-line medical consultation and therapy which conforms to social-distancing conventions. There is no contact and therefore no risk of transmitting the virus while looking after sick patients, whatever illness they might have. It sounds easy – just pick up the phone, talk to the patient and start your virtual consultation and treatment without even knowing who is on the other end of the line.

However, despite the nice-sounding name this process has been given – telehealth – it is not acceptable to my conscience. I believe firmly in the principle that a doctor should not make a diagnosis and treat their patient without a face-to-face chat to start with, and an appropriate physical examination if necessary. But telehealth has now become the norm and is in vogue and entrenched in the medical practice, and may well remain so until well after the world has recovered from the pandemic. And that will most likely not come about until an effective vaccine has become available on the market. So, what else could I do except retire, stop talking to patients, stop treating them too, and abandon my proud dream?

During the four stages of lock-down in Australia – this 'Lucky Country' was lucky because of the swift move to control the spread of the coronavirus ordered by Scott Morrison, our (brilliant) Prime Minister. The Australian Government carried out an effective programme of control after regular consultation with medical experts and heads of States, so that all in all Australia suffered very few deaths compared to other countries, a ripple in the pandemic sea against the tsunami figures of other countries like the US, Brazil and India. Approaching the end of 2021 Australia has suffered eighty deaths per million compared to the more than two thousand deaths per million in the USA, Italy, the UK and other advanced countries, while the toll is in excess of three thousand in many Eastern European and Latin countries.

In the lockdown months, the government has tried hard to inform people, console people, encourage people to register with COVIDSafe – the mobile phone tracking app, to work online, to exercise, to spend more time caring for their kids, and basically to inspire people to find something worthwhile to do to counteract depression, domestic violence and mental illness. In addition, the Government spent billions of dollars on the Jobseeker and Jobkeeper supplement payments to help workers keep their jobs, and the unemployed to survive, at least until the social and economic climate reasonably improved. That is what a smart and caring leader and government should do in this difficult time, to gather the support and cooperation of the nation's people.

Seeing now that I am a reluctant retiree, I must find something to kill the time with after my daily exercise. Fortunately, I have always been fascinated by the theme of living longer, but I have just never found enough time to pursue the topic while working full time in general medical practice, even though my limited knowledge, and my intuition, tells me that I could live longer because of my rather healthy lifestyle. My son David, who reads widely, has a good nose for sniffing out useful books, and has very helpfully been regularly sending me volume after volume on health-related topics. Younger generations these days are experts in on-line research and purchasing. David is no exception. He used to visit big downtown bookshops like Dymocks, but has shifted more and more to online ones like Amazon and The Book Depository. So as soon as I started to retreat to my bookshelves, I reconnected with my passionate interest – the topic of how to live longer.

After reading and studying a variety of texts, I was particularly thrilled by the one written by David Sinclair, a brilliant scientist and researcher on longevity, who used to be based at Harvard University's Paul F. Glenn Centre for the Biology of Ageing Research and is now based at University of New South Wales in Sydney. He operates and teaches on both continents, travelling to and fro like an "astronaut" – a term used with fondness by Hong Kong people to describe those husbands who fly regularly between HK and Australia (well, previously, since it's no longer possible due to the international travel ban in place in both countries).

Outline of this book

I will start first by giving the readers a general summary of some interesting facts and findings on many well-known demographics. These will be drawn from surveys of centenarians (people who live to one hundred years and beyond) in different regions in the world, with their vastly diverse ethnic backgrounds, interesting environments, favourite foods, eating habits, lifestyles, etc.

Following this, we will explore our body and systems, down to the cellular and subcellular levels to understand more how we live, function and resist all sorts of diseases, and how the body copes with major killers such as heart attacks (MI or CVD), diabetes mellitus (DM) and cancers in general.

Then, we will discuss the most exciting part of our journey to longevity – made more exciting by Professor David Sinclair's breakthrough discovery of a group of naturally occurring chemicals – enzymes – that can activate our body's 'longevity gene', also called the "vitality gene". All in all, once we factor in a few more key points, we will discover that it looks like living longer is not such an elusive dream after all. This hope, which seemed unreachable for human beings for centuries, may now be something right in front of us that can be put in our control, at least by most of us. That is what I want to share with you and for you to share with as many people as you can

Chapter Two: A Guided Tour of the World's Centenarian Blue Zones

Short lives until a short time ago

Looking back at the evolutionary tree of human life, you may be stunned by the very brief life spans of humans in the Bronze Age – the average being a mere eighteen years. In Julius Caesar's era, people died off at around twenty-teo years old, most of them dying from infections of all sorts. With improved hygiene, drinking water and sewage systems, things started to look up, and the life span then averaged from forty-seven to fifty-six and a half years.

This reminds me of the popular Chinese belief often expressed by many Hong Kong Chinese of the older generation that it is pretty rare for anyone to be able to live to seventy years old. It may be hard for us to realise that a mere seventy years was the maximum life span imaginable in China since ancient times. But then, the discovery of penicillin by Alexander Fleming in 1928 completely changed the picture, giving many more years' life to the average person. Life expectancy rose to between seventy-eight and eighty by around year 2000 and onward. The lesson we can learn here is that infection by germs and viruses have always been one of the deadliest enemies of health and has cut short untold multitudes of human lives.

The 2019 coronavirus pandemic is the latest reminder, infecting over thirty million people and killing close to one million. At the time of writing, it is still running rampant over many nations in a second wave and third wave and beyond, and this is expected to continue until suitable vaccinations have been carried out. After a fierce race to produce the first safe and effective one by over more than a hundred vaccine and infection control research centres, a few have been put into production, but not without controversy as to their safety and effectiveness. Disappointingly, whatever we tried, the WHO poured cold water over our heads by declaring in early 2021 that there would not be a guarantee of smooth sailing for many of us for decades to come. Okay, we certainly must try to follow the golden rules of social distancing and frequent hand washing and mask wearing on public transport and in crowded venues until the dust has settled properly. But all that aside, the fact remains that much progress has been made by science and medicine and as a result, our chances of living longer than ever before remain very high, even if we now have to factor in taking precautions against the coronavirus into account.

Blue Zones

Let us now turn to the adventures of a bunch of enthusiastic journalists, demographers, doctors and cardiologists from Australia, Canada, Hawaii, Japan, and the United States who together have shown us the five regions in the world famous for having the highest concentration of centenarians. These have been nick-named "Blue Zones" due to the fact that one of the demographers accompanying Dan Buettner (a longevity enthusiast and writer) used a blue pen to mark those areas in Sardinia denoting the highest concentration of people living to one hundred and over. So the term Blue Zones has since stuck as the new designation for regions with high concentrations of centenarians (people aged over one hundred semi-supercentenarians (those aged over one hundred and five), and super-centenarians (those aged more than one hundred and ten+).

Interestingly, the world's oldest person was the French woman Jeanne Calment who lived to one-hundred and twenty-two, while the oldest man on record is Bob Weighton who has just passed away in his home in the UK, aged one hundred and twelve, on 30 May 2020, and should qualify for the Guinness Book of Records provided his documents are verified.

The five Blue Zones visited and studied are:

A small town called Bapan, in the Bama county in the North-West of China, not far from the border of Vietnam.

Okinawa, a prefecture (state) of Japan, which is an archipelago consisting of one hundred and sixty one islands which lay between Japan and Taiwan.

Sardinia, a small island in the Mediterranean Sea, 120 miles west of Italy, with a small population of over one and a half million.

Loma Linda, meaning 'lovely hill' in Spanish, in California, USA, population twenty-one thousand.

Nicoya peninsula, off Costa Rica, in Central America.

Some of you may naturally wonder, with the world's population expanding and ageing, shouldn't there be more clusters of elderly people and centenarians? Well, there are: for example, the number of centenarians in Japan has increased to thirty thousand, and even Australia now has for thousand. However, nowhere else where reliable studies have been carried out can we find such significant clusters as in the abovementioned Blue Zone regions. The reliability of the studies carried out in Blue

Zones is guaranteed by the age of the subjects having been properly documented and verified to eliminate the possibility of deliberate deception, exaggeration and faulty memory.

Over the years, there have been a few areas whose claims were exaggerated because the local people liked to pretend to be older than they really were to gain more respect from their clan and society. Frequently, some sort of honour was received from their governments who felt a strange sense of pride at being able to show off the age of their citizens in the same way people parade expensive cars, houses or wealth. Here are a few more of the more well-known areas with long-lived populations:

The Caucasus mountain region in the former Soviet Union, covering the Georgia area which is the birthplace of Joseph Stalin. These people claimed to have fifty centenarians per one hundred thousand, which is a pretty high concentration of extremely long-lived people. They also announced to the world that yoghurt was one of their favourite foods and that it helped them to live longer. This greatly excited yoghurt production companies, and no doubt sent their production (and their shares) sky high.

However, when reporters, demographers and movie makers from all over the world flew in on their fact-finding missions, they were greatly disappointed as few claimants could produce bona fide birth certificates to show their true ages. In fact, there was no central birth and death registry until the Soviet Union was founded in 1917. After a more thorough analysis and investigation, most of the claims were found to be grossly exaggerated. This was for many reasons, including wanting to please Joseph Stalin who was born in Georgia.

The Hunza Valley of Pakistan did not fare much better, even though the environment offered people a sort of Shangri-la atmosphere which could be expected to help its inhabitants live more healthily and happily. However, while this is an important element for longevity, proof-of-age to support claims of longevity was problematic. They had no birth certificates and no health records and without either one, anyone in the village could exaggerate his or her age.

The last region of note is the Village of Vilcabamba in the Ecuadorian Andes, which proved to be among the most disappointing. Among eight hundred and nineteen villagers who were mostly elderly, not a single centenarian could be found by demographers.

However, the five previously listed official Blue Zones represent renowned clusters of centenarians, and have all been reliably checked by professional demographers and scientists, mostly through research into national birth and death registries and other available records.

Bapan: the longevity village, China

Now let us hear the incredible but real story of an American interventional cardiologist, Dr John Day, who in his prime at the age of forty-four decided to give up his busy lucrative practice in Utah as a pacemaker implantation specialist to move with his whole family to the remote, mountainous village of Bapan in China. He wished to learn how to improve his health and fitness so he could get back to his beloved marathon running and cardiac procedure practice. To many people, this story is too dramatic, too hard to believe, that this Johns Hopkins medical graduate who had trained in cardiac procedures at Stanford University was willing to sacrifice his busy practice and all the luxuries most Americans like: doughnuts, bagels and diet coke for breakfast, pizza and diet coke again for lunch, or cheeseburgers and fries and cookies for dinner (all of these unhealthy foods are prevalent in most US hospitals and are supplied free to busy doctors, interns, specialists and guest speakers). Who would think Dr Day would give up all he was used to, to move thousands of miles to live in an impoverished village? However, as unbelievable as it sounds, his move was absolutely logical and in the end, he was duly rewarded with a loss of weight, a return to normal good health and a happy family.

Initially, Dr Day had been very fit, having been a marathon runner for twenty years. But under the intense work pressure to increase productivity – a prevalent problem due to the work ethic in the US – he became used to working too many hours, taking too few vacations, and living on hospital food he himself called 'trash'. He became increasingly unfit and had high cholesterol and high blood pressure. He was overweight, suffered from insomnia and chest pain, and he was on six medications. In short, he was in very poor health. He was also absolutely disillusioned with his professional career and had an unhappy family life – he realised that he needed a drastic change.

Luckily, he had studied Mandarin, and he heard about this remote village in Quangxi province in the southwest of China, nick-named the Longevity Village. So his whole family moved there in 2012 and lived there for three months in order to learn their ways so that they could become healthy and happy again. Indeed, after living in the village, learning the local culture and habits and applying them himself for six months, he lost thirty pounds and his blood pressure and cholesterol were down to normal – really amazing! Most importantly, he felt more happy himself and went back to visit the village three times within two years. So now we will look at what Dr Day learned in the Longevity Village.

On the first day he was surprised, as well as partly disappointed, when he was shown how to make *longevity soup* with just some crushed hemp seeds and pumpkin greens. The result was not at all tasty compared to the doughnuts and cheeseburgers back in the home country. The woman who made the soup reassured the doctor that it was indeed a very simple soup and was served every morning. 'What else do you expect?' she said.

He met the oldest man of the village, whose confirmed date of birth was 1898, meaning that he was one hundred and fourteen years old. This old man was observed walking steadily to the fields to engage in farming on a daily basis. He was still his large family's main provider. Surely that is incredible! While most people somewhere between the ages of sixty to eighty are already limping or using a stick to walk, if they don't wind up sitting in a wheelchair and being pushed along by a carer in a nursing home, this 114-year-old not only manage to move about briskly, but was the main provider for his large family of children and grandchildren! The doctor was also shocked to see that this supercentenarian was exceptionally alert and physically agile, almost as much as people half of his age, and his body movements were as swift and effortless as the doctor's nine-year-old son. The villagers usually missed their breakfast to go down early to the field and worked all day for up to sixteen hours before going home for their dinner with the family. Such a lifestyle practice is not unlike the type of intermittent fasting or caloric restriction that has been upheld for centuries as the most consistent and effective factor for longevity. We will talk about this more in the longevity section.

In his diligent search for the secret of longevity in this village (population only about five hundred and fifty), Dr Day did some genetic tests on six of the seven centenarians. He detected that the majority of them had bad genes that predisposed them to cardiovascular diseases (CVD) like high blood pressure (HBP) and atrial fibrillation (AF) – a common form of irregular heartbeat, myocardial infarction (MI) – meaning heart attack, and some other diseases. He himself knew very well the prevalence of those serious diseases in the US, that the incidence of CVDs are seventeen times higher than in rural China, breast cancer is ten times more prevalent, and dementia more than three times as common. And yet these folks, young or old, had never had to consult a doctor – of course they had never had medical services anyway. Studies of those villagers over one hundred years old had found only four per cent with minor heart disease.

Another study of 267 villagers averaging eighty-eight years old had uncovered only one case of dementia; while in the US, eighty-five per cent of 85-year-olds have CVD and fifty per cent have dementia.

Could the longevity in this village be heritable and passed on to their children, grandchildren and great-great-grandchildren? A great many people these days are tempted to blame their 'faulty genes' on a lot of physical problems and mental illnesses which they often don't understand. But a well-known study in Denmark on three thousand identical twins showed clearly that longevity seemed only moderately heritable, about twenty-three per cent for males and twenty-six per cent for females.

So, could the villagers' diet be a significant contributor to their longevity? Quite possibly. The villagers are all hard workers and physically pretty tough, right from the time they are young children. They all eat good, healthy foods – greens harvested from the field or their garden plot, which are all fresh and full of nutrition, have never been refrigerated, and were never contaminated with chemicals and insecticides. Plenty of garden vegetables; wild fruits, plenty of root and tuber vegetables like sweet potatoes which are consumed at every meal; a good variety of grains, nuts, seeds and legumes. Meat is consumed in minimal amounts. They do not eat processed food, eat no sugar, no dairy foods like milk, cheese and cream, partly because there is no dairy farming, and partly because of their lactose intolerance.

He also noticed the villagers were contented, happy and smiling most of the time, and did not take any misfortune too seriously. Taking this sort of attitude would often add another eight years of life as concluded by a research study on a group of six hundred and sixty older Americans. We know that "laughter is the best medicine" and that anger and mental upset often increase your risk of CVD. This observation made Dr Day reflect on his suspicion that most doctors don't like their work of patient care. This is particularly relevant to psychiatrists, whose suicide rate is generally a few times higher than the general public's. Only about thirteen per cent of Americans like going to work, but they work harder and longer hours than most people in other developed countries: on average forty-seven hours with some working up to sixty hours per week.

The other tradition that caught his eye was that every house in the village had a special corner with a shrine decorated with food, often fruit, and their ancestors' pictures, showing that their parents were always remembered – a simple and effective way to remain connected. In addition, almost all of the villagers had their whole family gathered at every meal, in great contrast to Americans who it has been reported by the USDA Economic Research Service, spend half of their food dollars on fast foods which are consumed outside their homes. This practice of solitary eating has become twice as prevalent as it was in 1970. In the US, one in five meals is eaten in the car in the form of fast food through delivered through the windows. A minimal amount of vegetables accompanies these meals. One can only imagine how badly many Americans are connected to their families, their workplaces and communities. Feeling lonely and disconnected in any way often hatches the seeds of mental illness and poor health.

Dr Day, who was a pacemaker implantation specialist and spent a term as president of the Heart Rhythm Society, noted that atrial fibrillation (AF) is the most common form of abnormal heart rhythm, and in US centenarians, AF sufferers number about one in four or twenty-five per cent. In Europe it is half that, or one in eight. But in the Bapan county, Dr Day put the ratio at one in thirty-four! And he is convinced that this is mainly due to the people's healthy lifestyle, which is based on better food, including plenty of fresh vegetables, having a supportive community, staying active and connected, and drinking tea all the time. There is absolutely no cigarette smoking and no drug taking of any form.

He also jotted down what foods those centenarians usually eat and what nutrients they contain. These will be listed and compared with diets in other Blue Zones at the end of this book for easy reference.

Okinawa, the 'Galapagos of the East'

The Okinawa archipelago is a group of 161 islands situated between Japan and Taiwan. Its nickname "the Galapagos of the East" is a compliment which indicates its wonderful environment of palm-tree lined shores endowed with a rich array of fauna, flora and rainforest. It is inhabited by a cluster of the world's longest-lived people, who are happy and healthy. Researchers have discovered that it is described in ancient Chinese historical notes as 'the land of happy immortals'; a 'Shangri-la' or simply 'Paradise'.

Those islanders have been extensively and thoroughly studied. The research was begun in the 1970s by Dr Makato Suzuki, a cardiologist, geriatrician and professor at Ryukyu University, with the backing of both the Japanese and Okinawan authorities. Dr Suzuki was joined in 1994 by Canadian twin brothers Drs Bradley and Craig Wilcox, the former a gerontologist – a specialist on ageing patients – and the latter an anthropologist – a scientist researching human origins and development. Together, the trio interview and regularly carry out general check-ups with modern medical equipment. They have made many trips to follow up as well as adding new centenarians to their study for an impressive total number of six hundred. In the end, the trio produced a large volume of very interesting and impressive research in 2001 called 'The Okinawa Program' which is unique in the world in the sense that there will not be another similar survey of centenarians of such magnitude again, partially due to the lack of resources for this kind of scientific work, but also due to more and more restrictions being imposed by local governments to protect centenarians from unauthorised invasion of their privacy by journalists, salesmen, commercial interest groups, or even plain stickybeaks.

The Okinawa study is particularly reliable because there were no major problems regarding false or exaggerated claims of extended age, because every city and village has kept a family register system since 1879 when it was annexed by Japan.

The statistics for the centenarian population represent a stark contrast to those for Americans as shown in the following:

The number of centenarians is over four hundre in the population of 1.3 million, or thirty-five per one hundred thousand, while in the US the ratio is 5-ten per one hundred thousand. But the centenarians in Okinawa are still in robust health, being all physically active, healthy and independent; while in the West, by the age of seventy most people have already lost sixty per cent of their lung function, forty per cent of their liver and kidney function, fifteen-thirty per cent of the bone mass and thirty per cent of their muscle power.

When the Wilcox brothers first arrived in Okinawa, they came across an ancient copper bell which used to hang in the front of the castle where the king of the Ryukyus lived (Okinawa was originally called the kingdom of Ryukyus but the name was changed to Okinawa after it was annexed by Japan in 1879). The bell was cast in 1458 and bears an inscription in ancient Chinese which describes the Ryukyu kingdom as being located in a favourable position in the southern seas, being blessed with some of the wisdom of Korea and maintaining close relations with China and Japan. The inscription claims that it is the ideal land where the immortals live (Shangri-la, which in Chinese literally means 'paradise'). So, it looks like the long lifespan of the villagers was already well recognised by some ancient Chinese visitors.

Equipped with the full set of medical instruments, and with the assistance of an Okinawan-speaking nurse who they were lucky enough to find (few local centenarians spoke Japanese), the

Wilcoxes met their first centenarian, a sprightly man who they took to be about seventy and probably the centenarian's son, but who, to their surprise, turned out to be the centenarian they were looking for! The full check-up including an ECG (electrocardiogram, a common instrument used to check the heart) was all normal except for a first-degree heart block, which is fairly common for his age group and needs no treatment. When being informed of his check-up results, this centenarian exclaimed 'I am in perfect health!'. So, this centenarian had basically nothing wrong with his body after a hundred years' usage. And this amazing phenomenon seemed to apply to most of the centenarians the trio met during their research.

In general, the Okinawan centenarians had been observed to be lean, youthful-looking and energetic with low stress levels and surprisingly low rates of CVD and cancer, including the stomach cancer suffered by many Japanese. Their arteries were amazingly young and clean, meaning they had minimal plaque. Their blood tests showed low levels of cholesterol and homocysteine (both have a lot to do with heart attack). As a result, the Okinawans suffered eighty per cent fewer heart attacks than North Americans.

As we know, some types of cancer are hormone dependent, notably cancer of the breasts, the ovaries, the prostate and colon. Somehow these cancers, once initiated, will grow faster and spread if the body has higher level of hormones like oestrogen that feed the cancer cells. But Okinawans were found to have 80 per cent less of this type of cancer than North Americans. These incredibly low rates of heart disease and cancer can be attributed to the diet and lifestyle practised by the Okinawans throughout their whole lives. They were found to eat unrefined, low carb meals with lots of vegetables and fruits, but a minimal amount of dairy and land-animal meat. They don't smoke, and only imbibe some alcohol.

Okinawans love all sorts of physical activities. While only forty per cent of Americans participate in daily exercise to improve their bodies, the Okinawans were so used to physical activities that they just took it as the normal way of life. They have been seen not only working on the farm and in the garden, but also doing keep-fit exercises such as martial arts, traditional dances and aerobic and anaerobic movements to maintain flexibility. By practising wise eating habits combined with regular exercise, they maintain normal body weight as measured according to the body mass index (BMI). BMI is calculated by dividing the weight of a person by the square of their height, and is an accepted measure of whether that person is overweight or normal. BMI is normal if it is within twenty to twenty-five. Most Okinawan's BMI is usually about eighteen to twenty-two. As most of the island's inhabitants were so healthy, they hardly needed any tests, even ordinary X rays, not to mention CT, mammography, etc. If you asked them about prostate cancer, they would tell you "never heard of it".

After a full check-up of over six hundred centenarians and many other "youngsters", the trio finally concluded their key findings on the factors which define the world's longest-lived and healthiest human beings, grouping them under eleven categories:

Excellent arteries

As mentioned above, Okinawans have amazingly clean and young-looking arteries, with low levels of LDL (low density lipid or bad cholesterol) and homocysteine – both are by-products of animal proteins, and are usually the culprit causing heart attacks. Okinawans also are not interested in salty food like salty miso soup and are therefore able to maintain normal blood pressure. In addition to other factors listed below, it is not surprising that they have got the best heart health in the world, with the death rate from heart disease at eighteen per hundred thousand compared with a hundred deaths per hundred thousand in North America.

A low risk of hormone-dependent cancers

Compared with North Americans, Okinawans are at very low risk of developing hormone-dependent cancers like breast cancer and prostate cancer (eighty per cent less), or ovarian and colon cancers (under fifty per cent). The researchers feel that this has a lot to do with their healthy lifestyle: Okinawans practise caloric restriction (CR) which means eating less than a full meal: stopping when you are about eighty per cent full. Due to human and animal experiments, CR has been known for decades to be the most consistent way to assure longer life. The fascinating underlying mechanism responsible for this, which has only been established recently, will be discussed in later chapters.

A diet of veggies and fruit

The Okinawans' diet consists of an ample supply of fresh vegetables and fruits – these are healthy foods because they are full of polyphenols and carotenoids, anti-oxidants, vitamins, minerals and fibres (polyphenols include phytoestrogen or plant hormones, a group of SERM – Selective Estrogen Receptor Modulators, which are protective against those cancers mentioned above. They are estrogen receptor agonist/antagonists, a chemically diverse set of compounds that act on estrogen receptors in different organs such as the breasts, prostate, colon and bones (he anti-breast cancer drug, Tamoxifan, is one of them). They help block cancer cells from feeding on your cells. When cancer cells are cut off from nutrition, they die off and cannot spread. Hence the importance of a lifelong habit on plant-based food rather than animal meat. Besides, the high-fibre content in plants, combined with low GI food (Glycemic Index) is protective because it reduces insulin and insulin-like growth factors which stimulate cancer cell growth.

Fresh fish

The Okinawans, being so close to the sea, have no trouble including seafood on their menu. In fact, most of them eat fish more than three times a week, so that they have three times more omega-3 oil in their blood than Americans. Their fish are usually the fatty oily salmon, mackerel and tuna. And omega-3 oil is well-known for protecting against CVD.

Lean, fit bodies

Another two anti-cancer protective factors are sort of complimentary to each other: having a lean, fit body with an excellent BMI and physique due to daily physical work and exercise. Naturally the Okinawans' body fat has been found to be within the healthy range of ten to twenty for males and fifteen to thirty for females. Anyone can have their body fat measured these days by using a bioelectrical impedance analysis (BIA) weight scale.

Strong bones

Okinawans have strong bones. These days we know that our bones are not a rigid, inactive framework like the scaffolding you see outside of any building under construction. Our skeleton, in fact, is an active, busy structure constantly changing and remodelling, for better or for worse. We build up our bones from birth and their growth peaks in our twenties, and then continuously declines, depending on whether we have a high enough nutrient intake (especially calcium and sunlight/vitamin D) and healthy exercise of the weight-bearing type to serve as the main stimulus for bone growth. When the weight-bearing parts of our bones are weakened past a certain extent as measured by a bone-density machine (DEXA in Australia, DXA in the US), fracture may occur due to a simple fall or an innocent twist. The consequences can be serious for someone of advancing age, because an injury of that kind means hospital treatment and a long convalescence at best. If it is the femoral (thigh bone) which fractures, the patient needs an operation, but even after that they could still die within two years from complications.

The statistics discovered by Suzuki, Wilcox and Wilcox showed that Okinawans have twenty per cent fewer hip fractures (this type is nastier than a spine fracture) than mainland Japanese, who in turn have forty per cent fewer hip fractures than Americans. It has also been discovered that at the age of sixty-five, about twenty per cent of American females suffer fractures. The researchers' opinion was that, apart from the aforesaid protective factors of having plenty of sunshine and vitamin D from their wonderfully congenial subtropical environment, the Okinawans also have plenty of calcium in their hard drinking water. At the same time, the ubiquitous flavonoids in their daily diet of plants rich in natural oestrogens are protective not only of their CVD health, and against cancer, but also enhance their bone health.

Good brain health

Most Okinawans are found to have remarkable mental clarity, even at the age of one hundred. Of course, our concept of how the brain functions has changed over the last thirty years, ever since an ageing mouse's brain cells were found to grow and divide. In other words, we no longer think the number of brain cells is fixed. Instead, we see the brain as being capable of growing new brain cells so long as there is appropriate stimulation – that is what the much-discussed concept of "brain plasticity" is about. Put more colloquially: if you don't use it, you lose it. The healthy, CVD-protective food eaten by Okinawans helps to lower cholesterol and harmful homocysteine, keeping the arteries in the brain clean. They have also been found to have thirty per cent higher vitamin E levels than Americans. Vitamin E is a potent antioxidant and another of the protective factors against Alzheimer's disease.

Natural menopause

Because of a healthy lifestyle of consistent exercise and a rich supply of phytoestrogen (flavonoids), Okinawan women tend to have a smoother, easier and shorter oestrogen cycle, delayed onset of menarche (or "period") and the earlier onset of menopause. The flavonoids serve as a natural blocker of oestrogen receptors to protect sensitive organs like the breasts, ovaries, uterus (and prostate in men) and colon against oestrogen dependent cancers, yet selectively allow oestrogen to benefit their cardiovascular systems and their bones, due to a well-recognised group of SERM. Compared to similarly aged Americans, the Okinawan centenarians have been found to have high levels of all sex hormones (DHA from adrenal glands, oestrogens, testosterones and growth hormones). This is yet more proof that they are physiologically younger and display fewer markers of biological age.

Reduced free-radical damage

Free radicals are normal products derived from our cellular metabolism. Oxygen released during the process of metabolism happens in every cell in our body and can move around inside the cell, theoretically damaging the chromosome, the genes, or the mitochondria (the factory of the cell). It is further theorised that this leads to the long-term damage of cells or organs, mutation of genetic material, chronic disease, and eventually ageing. The older Okinawans have been found to have lower levels of free radicals in their blood than the younger ones. This is likely to be due to the higher intake of flavonoids, the practice of caloric restriction and regular exercise. But, please note, this theory about free radicals damaging our genome and has been questioned by experts recently and may have little to do with the 'longevity gene' and the reason why we age. We will look into this question in more depth in later chapters.

Excellent psychospiritual health

Personality testing has found Okinawans are generally optimistic, and don't easily become dejected by harsh physical environments, for example damage to crops from the cyclones which occur regularly in that part of the world. In April 1945, Okinawan villagers suffered particularly heavy casualties and untold devastation of their lands when the islands became inundated with brutal battles between the Japanese and US marines. They took the situation calmly, accepted their fate and tended not to become stressed easily, being demonstrably more relaxed and adaptable than the Japanese or North Americans. Researchers have found that the villagers operate on "Okinawan time", indicating a kind of "take it easy, don't worry, she will be right" attitude.

The society on the whole displays a strong, deep spirituality, and this is particularly evident among the female members of the society who act as its religious leaders. They are active in prayer and worship, resilient and rather dominant and confident. Particularly in the rural areas, there exists a strong support system and mutual support organisation known as "moai", which is quite similar to Japan's concept of the "socially cohesive society", and this could be part of the reason why Okinawa's oldest remain active and independent until their extreme old ages. The eldest women are usually chosen to be the leaders of their organised religion and carry out various duties such as managing life's fundamental issues like death, bereavement and other crisis situations that require a leaders' advice, counselling and ability to arrive at decisions. In other words, these elderly people are looked upon as pastors, priests and arbitrators of societal norms who provide wisdom and guidance to their communities. In return, they feel they are needed by their communities, and this may give them extra reason to living longer.

Integrative health care
Okinawans are adaptable and open-minded regarding both Eastern and Western approaches to health care. The island has a subtropical climate and is richly supplied with a large variety of medicinal herbs as well as edible nutrient-rich plants. They also have modern medical health institutions, so the islanders are really reaping the health benefits of both worlds. The situation is somewhat comparable to that enjoyed by people in Hong Kong and Japan where many demographic reports show the population appears to live longer than in the rest of the world. In fact, the latest report by the WHO has listed Hong Kong as number one for the average longest living people at eighty-eight and a half years; it has overtaken Japan for the last two years, quite likely

due to the benefits of their health care, which is a combination of both Eastern and Western approaches.

Sardinia

This small island, with a population of 1.6 million, is in the Mediterranean Sea about one hundred and twenty miles west of Italy. It has seen quite a few visitors coming and going, including the Australian investigative journalist Ben Hills, and the award-winning American writer and researcher Dan Buettner who was well funded by the National Geographic and supported by a team of specialists.

It was a remarkable personal adventure for Ben Hills and his photographer companion to travel over a thousand miles across Sardinia. They visited many small villages and towns, interviewing twenty-four centenarians in the process as they searched for the formula for longevity. They also had discussions with academics at the local university of Sassari about their findings, which drew on years of surveys. The island appears to have many unusual features, and the inhabitants, their lifestyle and their religious faith are quite unique, and distinct from those of Italy, the nation to which the island belongs.

Real Sardinians are typically shepherds who are very dependent on their sheep and goats. The country is similar to New Zealand, in so far as the number of sheep is just about double the number of people on the island. Most of them live in about fifteen small villages between Ogliastra and the Barbagia, and they have been found to have a high concentration of centenarians: thirty-seven per hundred thousand, which is twice as many as in the US. Even if it is not as many as in Okinawa, that was enough for it to be dubbed a "Blue Zone" by Dan Buettner's demographer.

Sardinia itself is actually one of the most impoverished parts of the "old" European Union. In many of the isolated small towns scattered in the Blue Zones, old poorly constructed houses are collapsing and the population is declining as many younger people leave the island to seek greener pastures overseas.

Traditionally, Sardinians have been somewhat reticent about descending to the coastal areas to live or to catch fish because of the danger from malaria infection, pirates and invading armies. Sardinians have therefore depended mainly on their sheep. The men work hard. They get up early and have some goat's milk, cheese and home-made pasta before herding their sheep up the mountain where they will graze all day. They drink more goat's milk and eat a homemade lunch to get them through the day before heading home for their dinner and a glass of Sardinian homemade wine called *Canonau*, which is pretty potent stuff.

Their favourite national dish is said to be their simple tomato sauce with pasta, together with milk, and their special homemade cheese which comes in a great variety – altogether there are about three hundred and fifty to four hundred different kinds – makes this island a sort of paradise for cheese lovers. Often a man's wife will bring him his lunch, walking for hours up the mountain trail to reach her husband. Most of the centenarians Ben Hill interviewed work all day and every day, sparing no time for education or hobbies. Work is their only activity. Most of them have their own plot where they grow their own vegetables and grapes and make their own very special wine. They have a winemaker who has just turned a hundred, but is still working hard on his teo hundred and fifty hectare vineyard to improve the quality of his produce. He has even been able to win prizes and export his better quality wine to make money. Naturally, he is probably best-known as the oldest wine maker in Italy – maybe even the world.

Consanguineous marriage is extremely common because of the geographic isolation from the outside world; and often the cousins from neighbouring villages marry, or even from next door. This does not seem to affect the community nor the family relationship at all. In fact, the family unit and its integrity are always of the utmost priority and is supported even when both members of a couple are over a hundred years old. This seems to be a logical necessity for survival in that harsh environment.

Many of the centenarians have a large family, typically five to seven children, and possibly twenty-six grandchildren, and twenty-seven great grandchildren. And it is a tradition that all centenarians are very well respected and well cared for by their children. Usually, it is the granddaughters who play the leading role in care, cook their grandparents' favourite dishes, or support them walking uphill. However, most of the centenarians are exceptionally tough and independent, having been shepherds all their lives – hard lives too. It is often not unusual to see a 108-year-old still struggling to climb up to the church every Sunday all by themself. They are even proud to have their centenarian priest regularly on duty in the local church in the town of Ovodda.

The university team has uncovered a couple of seemingly genetic defects in many centenarians. Firstly, many have G6PD deficiency – a hereditary condition in which the absence of the enzyme G6PD results in the breakdown of red blood cells, with this usually being due to ingestion of certain foods like fava beans or drugs like anti-malarials. Secondly, Sardinia has got the highest incidence of NIDDM (a kind of diabetes in the older age group) in Europe. How they acquired that sort of chronic medical condition is a bit of mystery when almost no one is known to consume many sweets, sugary drinks, desserts or any of the modern sweet junk foods. The interviewers' impression of the islanders' diet is that it is typically composed of goat's milk, cheese, pasta, bread, vegies, legumes and occasionally some meat. Sweets are never on their table. On the other hand, almost everyone enjoys a glass or two of wine at dinner (and you cannot rule out some shepherds bringing a bottle with them to the pasture to drink with their cheese and bread at lunch, as a habit). *Canonau,* their home-brewed red wine, is notoriously potent. It's made from the grapes of ancient vines and there is always some sugar in the wine, and alcohol itself can be converted into sugar by the liver. So that may be the cause of the NIDDM.

Another study has discovered that Sardinia did not have even a single centenarian until after 1950 when hygiene and nutrition had improved. Penicillin and antibiotics becoming available meant that infectious diseases were more easily cured. Infant mortality is significantly reduced and modern medicine has also doubtless played an important role in assisting the inhabitants in attaining a longer lifespan.

It has been observed that one of the reasons to account for the longer lifespan of the Sardinian shepherds is the character of the men, who are 'strong-willed, evincing high self-esteem and great stubbornness'. The ratio of males to females is unusual, it being one to one, compared to most other Blue Zones where females are generally longer lived with the ratio commonly being one to four. Besides the difference in personality traits though, in Sardinia the wife is usually the one to run the house and sort out all the domestic worries, including finances. Unfortunately, the tough, unyielding character of the inhabitants might also explain why one of the towns named Orgosolo is the infamous "murder capital" of Sardinia with well over two hundred kidnappings over a thirty-two-year period from 1960 to 1992, due to a long Mafia-style blood feud.

At one of the "shepherds' festivals", Ben Hills was invited to join in a feast of roasted whole lamb. The journalist discovered every shepherd carried a sharp knife, and he found himself wondering if the implement was carried to facilitate the slicing of meat or for when arguments broke out!

In 2002, the oldest centenarian in Sardinia, a man by the name of Todde who died just nineteen days short of his one-hundred-and-thirtieth birthday, was able to claim the title as the oldest man in the *Guinness Book of World Records*. He attributed his living to that age to the following factors:

- Never smoking
- Eating a healthy diet of goat's milk, cheese and vegies from the home garden

- Being honest
- Drinking a glass of good wine every night with pasta (he made his own)
- Praying daily to God
- Enjoying the caring support of his family in his twilight years

Sardinians usually practise CR by necessity and eat very little meat, though they do eat fish if available but no sausage or salami. And as far as a sense of purpose goes, protecting and supporting their own families is considered to be of the utmost important in their life.

Their diet and nutrition will be further analysed in the last chapter, bearing in mind that although Sardinia is a bona fide Mediterranean island, none of the centenarians partake of the traditional "Mediterranean Diet" – the healthy diet given a big thumbs-up by Western nutritionists, dietitians, scientists and health-fanatics – that has swept the world. Only one centenarian admitted to Ben Hills that he had "vaguely heard about it" – what an irony! It demonstrates that the magical title "Mediterranean" does not mean much – it is the daily healthy food you have consumed on a regular basis that matters.

Loma Linda,

This is a small community with a population of twenty-one thousand, including about nine thousand Seventh-Day Adventists, living in and around Loma Linda, which is only about ninety-six kilometres East of smog-shrouded Los Angeles – the second biggest city in the USA. The name Loma Linda means "lovely hill" in Spanish.

The Adventists lead the nation in life expectancy by sticking to the unique lifestyle required by their faith, which requires that there be no smoking, no alcohol, and that they avoid "unclean" foods such as pork. They are generally discouraged from eating any meat at all and avoid coffee, rich foods, and even spices. As a result, their lifespan has been estimated by epidemiologists to be seven years longer for males, and not quite four and a half years longer for females than the average in North America. The Adventists are not a homogeneous crowd – some are more strict about food than others and may fairly be called vegans. Strict vegans make up about four per cent of the group and enjoy lives that are up to ten years longer.

Because of their lifestyle, they have been included in two studies and surveys by the American Cancer Society, firstly, in 1974 in regard to the connection between smoking and lung cancer, and then in 2002 for a study of heart diseases and cancers.

Epidemiologists can now say with confidence that vegetables, fruits and whole grains seem protective against cancers; frequent meals of tomatoes reduce the risk of ovarian and prostate cancer by seventy per cent. The Adventists who eat meat had sixty-five per cent increased risk of bowel cancer, while those who ate more nuts and legumes had a forty per cent lower risk. These effects also appear to be relevant to pancreatic and bladder cancer.

This religious group has established their own university, hospital and church. The members are encouraged to observe the weekly sabbath. One pastor's opinion is that the sabbath serves as a stress reliever, at the same time making adherents feel connected and reinforced in their faith. Basically, the weekly service and day of rest is a sort of "sanctuary in time". This may possibly be another powerful factor in their living longer.

The conclusions drawn by epidemiologists on the secrets of longevity for the Seventh-Day Adventists in Loma Linda are not only locally indicative, but are also relevant to everyone who follows the regime of this religious group. The guiding principles are:

- Maintaining a healthy BMI (body mass index, or body weight in practice)
- Practising regular moderate exercise

- Having a day of rest, once a week, as a way of maintaining one's connection to others
- Spending time with like-minded friends (in this case, other Adventists)
- Doing voluntary work to help others less fortunate, for example through missionary service
- Sticking to their mainly vegetarian diet
- Having a light dinner early in the day
- Snacking on nuts

Costa Rica, Nicoya Peninsula

Costa Rica is a small country in Central America. It was well-known for being widely infested by malaria and dengue fever, and notorious for revolutions. So, for a long time their demography has not been fully surveyed, and their longevity has gone unnoticed. Certainly, little attention has been paid to the Nicoya Peninsula, one of the most isolated parts of Costa Rica for over four hundred years. Only recently has this area started to receive increased attention from the government, and now they have one of the best public health services in the region.

Dan Buettner's team attempted to map out the Blue Zone on the Nicoya Peninsula, an area first suspected to exist by one of the demographers from the University of Costa Rica. Unfortunately, due to on and off infestations, repeated revolutions and political instability, the data on the population has understandably never been as reliable as those in the better known and more politically stable regions like Okinawa and Loma Linda.

Still, with the help of many local academics and others, the team managed to round up a couple of dozens of advanced age groups, from ninety to a hundred years old, and carried out interviews and observations on their lifestyles and diet, and they came up with the following unusual features of this cluster of people.

On the whole, Nicoyans are mentally quite sharp, physically active, have strong work ethics and a zeal for family life. Sexual mores are exceptionally liberal, with many men appearing to have a relationship outside their marriage and quite often starting a new family in a different place, while their partner turns a blind eye. However, the women are not much more conservative, with a minority living with new partners. According to one of the academics who did approximately six hundred and fifty interviews, about seventy-five per cent of men have sex outside their marriage. A ninety-four-year-old man who went down to town every week to buy food to support his family of six casually mentioned that he also had two other kids by a village girl. He was observed to walk down the street twenty steps ahead of Dan Buettner when most people at that age cannot even get out of their wheelchair.

The Nicoyans are intelligent enough to embrace new health incentives from the government with open arms; they attend local clinics for any health problems and for recommended vaccinations. Their favourite foods are tortillas, a kind of corn or maize ground and turned into dough and cooked. Also popular are beans, rice, and plenty of fruits not only grown in their back yards, but also from the forest, including exotic varieties. These healthy natural foods allow them to benefit from their powerful anti-oxidants and phytoflavonoids (important nutrients from plants). That may explain why the Nicoyan incidence of stomach cancer is much lower than in neighbouring San Jose, even though children of both regions were found to be infected with Helicobacter pylori (the stomach bugs belonging to a genus of spiral flagellated Gram-negative bacteria found to be responsible for stomach inflammations, ulcers and cancers). This is possibly because the Nicoyan diet may have more cancer suppressing or cancer fighting polyphenols which are known to be more protective against cancer of the bowel, ovaries, breasts and prostate.

Chapter Three:
Reflections from the Centenarian Blue Zones Tours

After our grand tour of these Blue Zones, we have gathered enough reliable health and disease data from the studies for some conclusions to be drawn. The reader has already been given a good general impression of common factors in the lifestyles of centenarians and super-centenarians everywhere. These studies and statistics are extremely valuable because no one else would, for maybe up to another decade, be able to organise similar expeditions on such a large scale in terms of manpower and resources.

The travelogue offers us a macro picture of how these people can live so long and so well. We begin to understand how they remain disease-free most of the time, and even manage to avoid such major killers as cardiovascular disease and cancer.

So now let us list the dominant features common to most Blue Zones and centenarians.

The environment

The Blue Zones all seem to have favourable elements of their own that have quite likely given the inhabitants some advantages: for example, Bapan, the longevity village in China, has fertile farmland, an unpolluted river with clean running water filled with lots of healthy fish, and is isolated from the larger cities with their polluted air and motor cars. The villagers avoid factory-made products, an unhealthy diet and the kinds of junk food prevalent in the developed world. Their village has been preserved in its pristine rural state, pure and natural, for the last four hundred years. That is until recently, at least, according to Dr J Day, when Bapan started to change and become contaminated with a flood of junk foods, other unhealthy foods and drinks, modern amenities, and hundreds of health-seeking tourists and sticky beaks. This is all the result of the construction of a new direct road by the provincial government, perhaps made with good intentions, to open up this remote and badly neglected corner of China to the public, and to update local health facilities. Despite these recent changes, there is little doubt that a healthy natural environment has had a great influence on the villagers' mental and physical wellbeing. This is absolutely an important factor in prolonging lifespan.

Such beneficial effects are nowhere more obvious than in Okinawa – which is extolled as being a Shangri-la (*paradise* in Chinese). Indeed, this idyllic place creates the feeling within both inhabitants and visitors that one is virtually living in heaven. Such sensations themselves indirectly confer some subtle magical effect that benefits the brain, the heart and the immune system – the three most important factors directly involved in one's lifespan. It was no surprise that the visiting scientists were very well received. They found the centenarians extremely happy, polite and most helpful throughout the series of interviews. The exquisite subtropical climate with near-magical rainfall and pleasant humidity, along with plenty of sunshine, has gifted this archipelago's beautiful seashore with swaying palm trees and magnificent rainforests rich in flora and fauna. And the Okinawans are happy to spend all day, every day and every year, working in the fields and their garden plots, cultivating their nutritious greens, grains and tubers. There is absolutely no need for these elderly villagers to take the trouble to go downtown to buy unhealthy junk food, something which is foreign to them anyway. The raintree forest has provided a rich variety of medicinal herbs for the islanders to pick and use as natural remedies for their occasional health problems. So we can say that the congenial climate has created a congenial environment in Okinawa, which in turn has thoroughly infused every inhabitant in this paradise with the healthy and vitalising energy the Chinese refer to as chi.

You might think the environment could be a negative element for Sardinia – this rocky and impoverished island in the Mediterranean. However, it is not quite as bad as that, because, according to Ben Hills, most of the long-lived shepherds roam about on the top of plateaus, paddocks and mountains. The location affords the shepherds a vantage point on their way to work, downhill onto the seashores, from which they take in the panoramic views down below, described as "breath taking, extremely refreshing and exciting". It is certainly an enticement for any enterprising person to build a holiday villa or cottages for health-seeking tourists. Naturally, the clean, pure sea breeze on the mountain tops cannot be matched by the cities dotted along the coast.

When you come to look at Loma Linda, the American Blue Zone, the situation is very different. The area is sixty miles east of Los Angeles which is the second largest city in North America and notorious for its heavy smog due to its geographic situation: LA lies in a basin surrounded by deserts and mountains as high as ten thousand feet. With its population of nearly four million and tens of thousands of big motor cars on the city's busy highway network, it is not hard to see where the brown exhaust smoke settles – over the basin. The air quality in LA could not be much benefit to its people. In fact, the residents there could add another five to seven years to their lives if they breathed fresh, clean air every day like the Loma Linda people.

The Blue Zone in Central America represents a somewhat better picture, especially the Nicoya Peninsula, which has been one of the most isolated regions in Costa Rica for over four hundred years. Clearly it has not been contaminated by industrial nor commercial waste and the whole region remains pretty well a pristine natural environment for the local population to enjoy. The recent introduction of modern health services is another plus.

Physical work and exercise

From the descriptions and follow ups by all the scientists and journalists, no one could escape from the overall impression that almost all the centenarians have been hardworking folks ever since childhood. They get up at daybreak and start working in the field all day and every day until sunset, before returning home for their dinner, as happens in Bapan, the longevity village in south-west China, where Dr J Day met his first supercentenarian of a hundred and fourteen years old, doing hard manual work on the farm and still proud to be the main provider of his large family. It's really incredible. This has become such a stark contrast to the ridiculous situations in modern society in the West, in particular North America, where many people of seventy to eighty years old already have difficulty walking, and some cannot even get out of their wheelchairs! Why is there such a huge difference in people's mobility? Clearly the basic faults are in their eating and exercise habits (keeping in mind that less than forty per cent of North Americans regularly exercise). We will discuss diet, a sizeable topic, in another section of this book, after we take a good look at exercise routines.

You can recall of course the villagers in both Bapan and Okinawa have undergone check-ups by cardiologists, geriatricians (specialists for the elderly) and demographers who were really shocked that they could find nothing wrong medically with these people who had spent a hundred years working, digging and carrying heavy loads in the fields and on farms. The shepherds in Sardinia are physically not far from this in their daily ritual of getting their flock up and down the mountain seeking a better grazing field, or attending their garden plots with vineyards, vegetables and fruit trees for their families. Many brew their own special wine. Without the slightest doubt, the shepherds have to do a tremendous amount of walking which keeps them fit and healthy. As the ancient philosopher and physician Hippocrates said: "walking is the best medicine for mankind".

Unfortunately, we city dwellers have almost no hope of following this type of vigorous daily drill. We are mostly sedentary workers trapped in the unenviable cycle of working nine to five, Monday to Saturday, with a few valuable hours spent with either the family or the TV screen in a comfortable lounge chair doing nothing – because we are tired, or we have had enough stress at work.

However, you can modify your lifestyle to some extent and exercise hard and train your body, like Marge, aged a hundred, in Loma Linda's Seventh-Day Adventist compound. She begins her day with a mile walk, an exercise-bicycle ride, and some weightlifting. She recounted her story to Dan Buettner while doing thirty mph on a bike non-stop. So like all these admirable centenarians, you should try your best to keep your body moving, lubricating and churning, whether walking outside, riding an exercise bike, or working out on a rowing machine, practising Tai Chi or just doing some all-round stretching. Many studies from all over the world will show you that simple exercises can re-boot your CVD and your energy system so that after a while on a regular exercise regime, you have more energy left after work to play with your kids or do household chores and the weekend gardening.

Exercising to keep fit and healthy has been one of the lynchpins and main themes strongly recommended in my book *Total Health and Fitness Revolution* (readers can find it on Amazon online).

Dr Joseph Cheung

Being part of a community

Human beings are by nature social animals. They support their families and in turn need support from them. The heads of the family work hard to raise their offspring to be decent members of society, and in turn seek to be fully respected and loved by these family members and be taken care of in their twilight years. This has been an unspoken rule generation after generation since humans first appeared on earth and prospered. In the Bapan village, Dr Day's keen eyes observed that every villager's home had a special shrine decorated with their ancestors' pictures or photos. They burn incense there to show that family links always remain connected. In a way this practice also serves as a stabilising force and an aid to spiritual and psychological wellbeing. This family support and connectedness appears to spread through the entire village and you can see that neighbours, and even distant villagers, will come over to give a helping hand in building a shed, hut, or a house when a newcomer is in difficulty. This is community spirit and support at its best. These ideals are reflected in the wise Chinese saying, "store up grain for hunger, bring up children for old age".

In Sardinia, the family unit is equally strong and is regarded as the most important element in life by the shepherd. So, commonly the centenarian is very much revered, not only by his or her family members who pamper them and cater to all of their needs, but also by the whole community.

In one example of this, in the cold and wind-swept village of Arzana, the entire town prepared a festival to celebrate the hundred and ninth birthday of a semi-supercentenarian, one of the very rare people who have lived through three centuries. Even though the poor and declining town is not much to see and talk about, everyone got excited. The local school choir rehearsed a special song composed for that occasion, and the local florist organised a floral arrangement for the local church hall. Reporters and TV crews came in from out of town, building up the atmosphere like it was a festival. In the end, the petite birthday girl was ushered into the church hall with her GP on one arm and the mayor on the other, amid the excitement and the shrill cheering of two hundred village kids. There was a large birthday cake and candles, ribbons and banners. All in all, it was an extremely moving celebratory occasion showing how supportive those villagers are and how seriously they take showing respect for their senior citizens. Such feelings of being loved and looked up to without question definitely add a powerful impetus to the desire to live longer.

The Okinawans are basically quite similar in maintaining their family ties to their ancestors by reserving a secluded area in the house for their prayers for fortune, good health and protection. They are known to carry out such rituals daily. But there they have this tacit traditional idea that the oldest female member of the family will usually assume the role of a sort of religious leader in the community, performing prayers and conducting worship during social and celebratory gatherings. This encourages her to be more assertive and confident, and creates a feeling of being needed in the society. Often, they will form a smaller group of elderly people with similar interests who regularly meet at their houses to chat and discuss any matters of concern. It appears to scientists that they enjoy these small group chats tremendously, as these occasions function as an excellent way to remain connected to their friends and fellow villagers.

The elderly Seventh-Day Adventist members, on the other hand, experience smooth sailing right from the start, being followers of a strict religious tradition which encourages its members to do regular moderate exercise, attend the Sabbath, and communicate with members with similar interests. Adventist communities are set up to take care of their members, and most Adventists live in the area where they have their own university, well-equipped hospitals, gyms, and independent villa units for convenience. Therefore, without hesitation, Dan Buettner voted Loma Linda as the leading Blue Zone in North America, producing the highest concentration of centenarians due largely to their strong discipline, connectedness to their faith/religion, healthy diet, regular exercise, and generally having peace of mind, knowing very well they can get help and reassurance physically and mentally when needed.

Being free of anxiety and stress

Scientists visiting the Blue Zones are extremely impressed by the stress-and-anxiety-free lifestyle of the centenarians. Generally, in Japan, like in America, everything has to be on time and precise, and this creates a lot of stress and anxiety. In modern competitive societies, GADs (generalised anxiety disorders) are common. Over four million American males and twice as many females suffer from this malaise. A large part of this phenomena could be blamed on daily breaking news on TV screen showing violence, killings, flooding and catastrophic disasters such as bush fires and widely destructive tornados which result in hundreds of homes and properties being wiped out. Add to this the thousands of homeless and desperate people and the result is a general overload of negative information. It certainly doesn't help that feelings of wellbeing are associated with having to earn a living according to the American work ethic of trying to get every job done under restrictive time constraints. It is a telling fact that only about thirteen per cent of Americans like going to work. When pressure has built up for longer time, it results in chronic stress which can damage the immune system, causing many kinds of disease which influence lifespan both directly and indirectly (we will discuss this phenomenon further in another section of this book).

Fortunately, centenarians appear to be quite adaptive, and by readily accepting change are better able to avoid becoming stressed. They have their own agenda – not to rush, but to take it easy, like the "Okinawa time" practised on the Okinawa Islands, or the siesta taken by the Sardinians during the nearly three-hour break at lunch time. Ben Hills stated that he and his photographer were unable to find any shops open from noon to 3 pm, while locals observed their siesta time.

Centenarians are often described as possessing a uniquely cheerful personality full of self-confidence. They have good coping skills and are creative, independent and calm. Open, sociable and agreeable, these individuals also display a high degree of tolerance for frustration. All this contributes to their being optimistic people, which gives them a powerful immune system and therefore a much-extended lifespan.

One interview with an Okinawan (aged a hundred and one at the time, but destined to live on to reach a hundred and ten) revealed that he had suffered a great deal of hardship and uncertainty upon emigrating to Canada, but he wanted to share his secrets of longevity. His heartfelt advice was as follows: "[it is] important to have a good night's sleep. Never worry about little things, or age, or appearance, aches and pains; focus [on the] good things in life, and remember to smile". Not surprisingly, Jeanne Calment, the world's longest-lived person, reportedly offered essentially the same advice.

In other words, one should constantly remind oneself to maintain inner optimism and happiness – come what may.

Chapter Four: Longevity is Beckoning

Tales of searching for the Fountain of Youth

Eternal life seems to be the common wish of all humanity. One of the world's oldest written works, *The Epic of Gilgamesh,* tells of the King of the ancient realm of Mesopotamia and his quest for immortality. And "long live the King!" is the wish expressed by the nation to their beloved sovereign.

In the East, the mentality of all the Chinese emperors of every dynasty was no different. They had to be addressed as *Wan Shui*, meaning "ten thousand years of reign". Legend has it that the first Chinese emperor, Ch'in Shih Huang (259-210 BC) was a highly intelligent but merciless man, full of brilliant plans and wonderful foresight. He had become emperor at the age of only thirteen and started to manipulate and conquer the other six kingdoms, one by one, and in that way China was unified. In fact, the name "China" used in the West is derived from the name of Emperor Chi'in. Even at the age of thirteen, he had already dreamed of an eternal life as emperor, and started to construct the grand burial place in Si Ann with a splendour and magnificence the world had never seen before. The burial site, which covers fifty-six square kilometres, is recognised as the largest in the world, and was found to contain an underground palace hiding a copper coffin surrounded by mercury symbolising running rivers, while stone officials were placed all around to protect the palace, along with a complete army of over a few thousand life-size soldiers, chariots and generals, all skilfully crafted by stonemasons. The site is also known to have booby traps designed to deter cemetery diggers and coffin robbers.

The whole complex is simply amazing and based upon the out-of this-world idea that the young emperor had to enjoy his after-life as the ruling emperor in the sumptuous and protected underground palace. The area has been named one of the ten most iconic scenic places tourists must see.

In the emperor's obsessive search for the secret of eternal life, he heard about some magical plant that could prolong his existence. One of his eunuchs had offered to lead a team of five hundred innocent virgin children to the legendary mountain to find the plant which was supposedly located somewhere near the Korean peninsula. The expedition was launched amid pompous ceremony, but the ship never came back – legend has it that it set sail to Japan where its passengers set up their own territory.

There is another widely known story of searching for magical eternity – the Fountain of Youth – the fabled spring of water that could make people younger and bestow long life. It started with a Spanish explorer and governor of Puerto Rico, Juan Ponce De León, in the sixteenth century. He was said to have been exploring the northeast coast of Florida in April 1513 looking for the fabled fountain. As it was, he was injured in a skirmish with the indigenous people and died at sixty-one.

Given the never-ending desire to cheat death it is not surprising that there have also been a number of charlatans who promoted their own "Elixir of Youth". One famous case is that of a Doctor Paul Neihans who in the 1930s was operating in the La Prairie clinic on the shores of Lake Geneva in Switzerland. He promoted his elixir of foetal lamb and liver cells in injections which were delivered into the buttock of his clients which included celebrities like Charlie Chaplain, Marlene Dietrich and Pope Pius XII. However, there doesn't seem to be any evidence that this treatment made any difference to the longevity of the patients, though it doubtless made Dr Neihans' bank balance a lot healthier.

A doctor in Romania developed a "gerovital" injection course with the promise of curing peptic ulcers, osteoarthritis, Alzheimer's disease and multiple sclerosis etc. One of the shepherds in Sardinia tried this remedy for one month without any effect and declared the miracle cure no help at all. It was later discovered that the injection was just ordinary anaesthetic used by the dentist to numb pain.

In the late nineteenth century, a French physiologist, Brown-Seguard, promised long life with his formula of injections prepared from the testicles of guinea pigs and dogs! Again, the reality didn't live up to the hype. Another of these strange products purported to gift people with a longer life is from the Austrian doctor Eugene Steinach who promoted vasectomy as a way of re-vitalising sexual function.

The human appetite for longer life, however, has never abated, even though numerous charlatans, fools and crooks have come and gone after their bizarre claims were exposed time and time again. More recently, in 2002, some dozens of the world's longevity experts stated in serious tones that nothing in the world at that time could achieve anything in influencing the process of ageing. That was a very disappointing statement, and, in my view, an unfortunately short-sighted one, to say the least. And now we are in year 2022, and the world has steadily advanced in the search for such an elixir. Let us then discuss 2020, only two years past and a tumultuous year, before we trace back numerous studies and discoveries relevant to ageing and its secrets that have been occluded from the human race for decades or even centuries.

The year 2020 – a tumultuous year

The year 2020 was fundamentally a year of global catastrophe thanks to the COVID-19 pandemic: the "once-in-a-hundred-year event". Right from the beginning of the year, the coronavirus which is thought to be a variant of the SARS virus that raged across Hong Kong and SE China ten years ago swept through every nation on earth, infecting over eighty-two million people by the end of 2020.

Australia performed well in terms of dealing with the crisis, apart from the state of Victoria due to mistakes in hotel quarantine, applying the wrong strategy and misinterpreting the set infection-control model. Victoria became deeply trapped in its 2nd wave before requesting urgent assistance from the federal government.

But at the same time, throughout Australia during the hot summer months, large tracts of rural land and numerous townships were ablaze as near-uncontrollable bush fires swept across the nation. Hundreds of homes, towns and farms were destroyed and a number of human lives were lost in the devastation, as well as those of millions of native animals. Miraculously, after weeks with no apparent end in sight, the widespread firestorm was suddenly extinguished within days by a timely deluge, and peace returned to the suffering communities.

That was certainly a double whammy to the Australian economy with the travel industry badly mauled, and many small businesses collapsing or simply disappearing. The government of the day swiftly produced many rescue packages for most kinds of workers who had lost their jobs or were unable to pay their mortgages etc. One of the options was allowing people to withdraw money from their super funds for personal use to get over the crisis – a sensible and timely strategy. It is useful to recall that a future fund had been set up over ten years ago for future unfunded super pay-outs in a smart move from the then treasurer Peter Costello – the longest serving treasurer in Australian history – while John Howard was the prime minister. The fund had only sixteen billion dollars at the time, but by 2021 it topped out at a hundred and seventy-one billion due to clever investment strategies. This smart policy would prove a boon to the Australian people.

When summer arrived in the USA that year, in what was clearly no coincidence, exactly the same sort of wild bush fires started in California, and raged furiously over three states on the west coast due to the exceptionally hot summer and high temperatures which turned many towns and regions into infernos.

Then, a one-in-a-million accident happened in the beautiful city of Beirut on the 3rd of August when a stockpile of twenty-five thousand tonnes of explosive chemicals which had been stored for many years, in spite of protests from nearby householders, in a warehouse at the port not far from the city centre allegedly ignited out of the blue, causing a gigantic explosion, not unlike a mini atomic bomb. The force was so powerful that practically all surrounding buildings and houses were completely destroyed. The toll? A hundred and ninety-one dead, six thousand injured, and three hundred thousand homeless!

Yet another disaster occurred, this time on a Greek island when a fire swept through a refugee camp housing mainly Middle-Eastern refugees, causing twelve thousand people to become homeless.

So you can see all the governments and authorities concerned, including WHO and refugee services, were working non-stop with planning, delivering emergency foods and medicine, and setting up new camps and re-grouping refugees. What a year 2020 was. When we remember the civil unrest around the Black Lives Matter protests and anti-covid demonstrations, it might seem as though there was nothing but disasters and catastrophes, trouble and tragedy.

However, despite all this commotion and calamity, there has fortunately been steady progress made along the path to the Fountain of Youth, thanks to the dedication and conviction of hundreds of thousands of hard-working scientists who have been labouring for decades all over the world. Like everything else enshrined in mystery, we may gain some illumination if we consider some historical developments that started off quietly, and slowly built to a pinnacle in 2020. The solution to this elusive mystery has connotations for a wide range of sciences. Not only has it received the dedicated attention of scientists such as biologists, physiologists, geneticists and gerontologists that one might expect to have been involved in such a study, but it has also attracted immense interest from newer specialists such as molecular and evolutionary biologists, and immunopathologists (specialists in immune-system diseases). The result is, as you can imagine, that the study of ageing has come to incorporate a dizzying variety of theories and a huge phenomenological literature. In this book, we focus on a few well-known ones for insight.

Chapter Five: Knocking on the Door of Longevity

Historical notes

Nearly five hundred years ago, a Venetian nobleman called Luigi Cornaro published what was quite possibly the first book on longevity, titled *First Discourse on the Temperate Life*. The author wrote his discourse when he was in his eighties and he died in 1566 at nearly a hundred years old, which was clearly unusual in that era when the average lifespan was under forty. This chap had discovered some helpful ways of living a healthier lifestyle and in fact his diet and drinking habits were well documented: he ate no more than three hundred and forty grams of food and drank two glasses of wine each day "always leaving the table well able to take more". Clearly, he had found the common key to longevity – calorie restriction (CR).

Since then, there have been a few scientific experiments on rats exploring the effects of CR on lifespan, such as the one started just after World War I by Lafayette Mendel and Thomas Osborne – the duo who discovered vitamin A. They discovered rats on CR lived much longer than well-fed ones.

Following this clue, in 1935, Professor Clive McCay of Cornell University demonstrated that rats fed twenty per cent less food lived significantly longer than those fed on a typical lab diet. Studies from then on showed again and again a CR diet results in longevity for all forms of life.

In 1952, Sir Peter Madawar, a British immunologist, famed as "one of the most influential fathers of evolutionary ageing", proposed his theory of mutation accumulation, in which he postulated that ageing was caused by DNA damage resulting in the loss of genetic information, and by random mutations causing ageing characteristics. In other words, Madawar theorised that such DNA damage would be repeatedly copied at every cell division, building up more and more faulty DNA and genes, thus accelerating the ageing process. Nevertheless, this theory did not sound convincing a few years later when one of his co-authors, Leo Szilard, discovered how to clone a human cell. Following this, Keith Campbell at the University of Edinburgh successfully cloned the famous Dolly the sheep from an old cell; this became sensational news all over the world, proving that mutation of DNA does not cause ageing. If old cells had indeed lost vital genetic information in the damaged DNA, and that was the cause of ageing, we should not be able to clone new animals from old individuals with damaged ageing DNA – clones would be born old. Even though Dolly only enjoyed a short span of life due to the fact that she contracted a lung disease, the autopsy did not find any signs of ageing, refuting the misconception that clones would suffer premature ageing and die young. In fact, subsequent clones of pigs and sheep developed normally with normal lifespans.

In 1956, the "Free Radical Theory of Ageing" was proposed by Denham Harman, an American chemist and a founder of the American Ageing Association (now the American Academy of Anti-Ageing Medicine, or A5M). This theory proposes that free oxidants with unpaired electrons produced in a cell as part of the metabolic process were capable of inflicting damage on DNA and mitochondria. This harm is generally known as oxidative damage even though the oxidants are not confined to oxygen; they could be peroxide or hydroxide. Oxidants are produced in our cells continuously as part of the cellular metabolism so you can imagine there is some pretty intense activity happening in mitochondria, which is why it is often called 'the cell's powerhouse' due to its vital function of breaking down nutrients to produce energy. It also plays a major role in the battle between the immune defence cells (phagocytes) and invading viruses from colds, flus and infections. In addition, oxidants are also produced when the body is exposed to harmful external forces such as UV radiation, X-rays, pollution, tobacco, harmful chemicals, fumes from motor vehicles and household sprays.

Professor Lester Packer of the University of California, which is famed for being the world's leading antioxidant research centre, postulated that oxidants are effectively neutralised by enzymes and antioxidants produced in the body. Normally, people have five major antioxidants which form a network, consisting of co-enzyme Q10, vitamins C and E, glutathione and lipoic acid. With the exception of glutathione, all of these are sourced from foods and particularly vegetables and fruits which are rich in substances called polyphenols, isothiocyanates and carotenoids. Each one of them helps boost each other's power to control free radicals and protect the heart against CVD.

Over time, however, this theory was found to stand on ever shakier ground as numerous studies and experiments failed to provide proof of a decisive benefit of various antioxidants on controlling ageing. Most researchers consider the theory as having been overturned nearly ten years ago. Science has since demonstrated that the achievable health effects from an antioxidant-rich diet are more likely due to their stimulation of the body's natural defences against ageing which is achieved by boosting the body's enzymes that neutralise free radicals.

In 1998, Kenneth B Beckman reviewed major research literature on the study of ageing, and formed the opinion on Harman's "free radical theory" that although it has not been able to positively tackle degenerative senescence (ageing) head-on, it could contribute to explaining the ageing-associated stress of pathophysiology, the study of disease processes and their effects on the body, particularly to the immune system, and possibly the energy power house in mitochondria. These are full of enzymes

– up to a few hundred – and could be worn out as a result of exceptionally busy repair work on DNA damage. Mitochondria dysfunction is one of the signs of ageing, and a strong healthy antioxidant supply could ameliorate the distress and therefore be beneficial. They may not help that much while you are young, healthy and energetic, but could contribute some defence to your immune system against advanced ageing.

The latest and the most sensational finding of all was contributed by Professor David Sinclair, a molecular geneticist and director of the famous Paul Glenn Centre for the Biology of Ageing Research at Harvard. He stunned the world in 2002 with his discovery of resveratrol, a kind of plant phenol, which is one of several thousand types of substances collectively named polyphenols, flavonoids, or phytonutrients. Resveratrol can be extracted from many colourful plants and fruits, particularly from the skin of red grapes, especially from stressed plants; this small molecule and some others had been proven to turn on the longevity gene or the vitality gene. In the following year, 2006, he and Joseph Baur published their findings in the prestigious journal *Nature* detailing their experiments on mice, which proved that resveratrol-fed animals were well protected from CVD, NIDDM and Alzheimer's disease, and lived longer even without the help of CR and exercise. This news made international headlines as the world woke up to the incredible reality that a longer lifespan was no longer a mirage, but something we could tackle, something we could control, with some polyphenol from the plant kingdom.

But please note, we will be talking more about Resveratrol as a simple chemical able to activate sirtuin, the longevity gene, and there will be further elaboration as we go along.

Basically what Professor Sinclair presents in his theory on ageing is that ageing is not just a matter of getting older with all the degenerative signs of senescence like coronary heart disease (CHD), cancers, diabetes or osteoarthritis (OA); instead, he is convinced *ageing is a disease*, which occurs due to a loss of information at the subcellular level. Like heart disease and cancers, ageing can be controlled, retarded, or even somewhat pushed back to confer more healthy years of life to people.

His research and experiments on lab animals over the last 25 years have been a powerful foundation on which he has built up his concepts, his visions, and his theory, and he has reached his final goal. We will explore his theory and concept in further detail in another section of this book.

Navigating road blocks on the path to longevity

It is interesting to find out that lifespan can vary tremendously from one species to another, even though we are able to trace our genes all the way back to a primordial organism that first appeared about four billion years ago after the Earth was formed. So you and I, your pet dog and cat, the ferocious tiger and lion, the killer crocodile and shark, the mighty elephant, the majestic giraffe and every other living creature down to lowly bacteria, moulds and yeast are related. Isn't this incredible? Now let's take a look at various lifespans of some of them.

The lowly one-cell yeast – the base organism picked by D. Sinclair for many of his studies on ageing – lives about three weeks only. Gastrotrich, a minute sea creature, lives only three days. Conversely, giant tortoises can live for a hundred and seventy years. The bowhead whale in Alaska has been known to live for up to two hundred and twelve years. And Greenland sharks have been estimated to have lived more than five hundred and ten years! On another note, some jellyfish can detach part of their body and regenerate a new one.

But the plant kingdom members usually have a much longer lifespan. The oldest organic creature on earth is, in fact, the famous bristlecone pine tree of California. Some of the oldest are estimated to be over five thousand years old. Many spectacular pine trees in China's majestic mountains, for example Yellow Mountain, are known to be over several hundred years old.

There are many legends of long-lived people throughout history, but since birth certificates have been introduced there is no need to rely on hearsay. The longest-lived person in history is the French woman Jeanne Calment, who didn't pass away until she was a hundred and twenty-two, beating even the legendary Moses by two years. She recommended walking for exercise and two glasses of red wine daily. Her life seems to confirm the reality of the "French Paradox". This phrase was coined by French scientist Sege Renaud, whose famous scientific study conducted in 1991 led him to conclude that French people have a lower rate of heart attacks than most people in the West, even though they consume more high cholesterol food, because they drink wine regularly and consume 'good fats' rather than the unhealthy ones favoured by many Americans.

The human quest for longer life is as old as civilisation, and we have made quite some progress in that regard. During Julius Caesar's rule in the first century B.C., the average lifespan was twenty-two years, but by 2020 it had risen to eighty-five for woman at least, while in as recently as 1960 the average was twenty years younger than that.

Can we live longer still in the near future? Some scientists have maintained a rather pessimistic opinion on this. For instance, in 1990, Professor M. Little of Sydney suggested that even if all cancers were eliminated, the average human lifespan would increase by only a few years. This viewpoint echoed the general view of many biologists at the time that, in general, human cells could last no longer than ninety years. And, as recently as 2002, the world's longevity experts jointly declared that nothing could be done to influence ageing, meaning in a practical sense that people would die before eighty-five. A popular sentiment was that this was just "the way it goes", that it was "better for the society", and "young people should be allowed to take their place" – kind of a defeatist mentality.

Dr Joseph Cheung

However, a couple of decades on and none of those gloomy views have stood the test of time. Now the general consensus is that there is no such gene as an ageing gene - this consensus, together with D Sinclair's theory that 'ageing is a disease', has become the very important and fundamental basis for current researchers globally to work on in order to uncover the secrets of longevity. Our genes did not evolve to cause ageing; however, they do evolve constantly to improve our immune system so that it can fend off harmful invasive pathogens and manage the repair of damaged DNA. Ageing now is treated not as an inevitable degenerative condition, but rather as a disease that can be delayed, modified or even slowly reversed to give you a younger look and longer life.

Nonetheless, there are many significant obstacles and risks that may harm or shorten your life and block your path to a longer lifespan, so obviously anyone who wishes to live longer must prepare well to avoid these risks. Let's look at the major diseases (CVD and stroke) and cancers that could shorten your life, and tackle them one by one, allowing you to live a longer and healthier life.

Avoid a broken heart

As everyone who has experienced a broken heart or witnessed its impact knows, such an event can be one of the most devastating things that can befall a human being. It often leads to severe emotional upset, extreme depression and may even result in suicide. Medically speaking, however, when we talk about damage to your heart, we of course mean something more physical - CVD (cardiovascular diseases).The heart is an amazing organ which works day in and day out, twenty-four hours a day, seven days a week to keep us going. It beats one hundred thousand times a day, or thirty-five million times a year, never taking a break nor any sick leave (and if it does, of course, that means the end of your life). But a few things can go wrong if it is not well looked after, particularly if anything affects the blood supply moving through the coronary arteries, the valves, or its beating rhythms (the electrical system). Then there can be disastrous results such as myocardial infarction (MI or heart attack), congestive heart failure (CHF) or atrial fibrillation (AF).

Worldwide, MI tops the list of deadly diseases. In 2003, it was responsible for twenty-eight per cent of all deaths in the USA, or six hundred and eighty-five thousand deaths. In Australia, during the same time, it chalked up forty per cent of deaths (ten thousand). People in Okinawa, one of the Blue Zones, experienced MI at only eighteen per cent of the American death rate. Americans are certainly suffering poor heart health, reporting three thousand MIs per day. This rate is seventeen times the rate suffered in China, and obviously unacceptably high.

After the Korean War in 1950 when three hundred deceased American soldiers were autopsied, a staggering seventy-seven per cent of them showed gross evidence of CVD. This is in supposedly fit young soldiers! In a 1955 survey, the USA topped the twenty-odd countries included when it came to the number of deaths from MI. Since then, the number has dropped to fifty-eight per cent due to the development of modern cardiac surgical techniques like CABG (by-pass), stenting (the insertion of wire springs to keep blocked arteries open), and pacemakers. Even so, right now in the USA, about two thousand persons die of heart attack every twenty-four hours, far exceeding the maximum daily death toll of Americans (a thousand plus) during the COVID-19 pandemic.

So what kind of strategy should you choose to prevent a heart attack? This should be the most pressing question on everyone's mind and has become the most burning medical topic, not only in medical literature, but in hospitals, medical consultations in general practice, on current social media and on TV Q and A shows.

Now everybody knows "prevention is better than the cure". This simple principle, unequivocally, applies to heart attack much more vitally than to any other diseases. Currently, over the last few decades, the prevailing view as embraced by most enlightened family doctors and cardiologists alike is to adopt a healthier lifestyle.

However, not everyone is interested in a healthy lifestyle, nor able to follow one, because it requires a change in habits on a lot of fronts. Many people struggle to adopt stricter discipline and practise it for the rest of their lives, or at least for most of the time. For instance, many smokers refuse to quit smoking until they start to notice worrying symptoms like coughing up blood, and they become alarmed when their GP finds a large cancer on their chest X-ray. For those who cannot control their impulses, many useful and effective CVD drugs can be taken to treat hypercholesterolaemia and hypertension – the two major culprits leading to MI and CHF. But medications are not always one hundred per cent safe nor do they guarantee success. You need to see your GP for a regular check and adjustment, to make sure that the medications prescribed are effective in lowering your BP (blood pressure) and blood lipids (the cholesterol).

Importantly, your GP will make sure you are not overtreated for HBP causing your BP to go too low, which can result in dizziness and weakness. They should also ensure that you are not allergic to any of the drugs prescribed. For example, the bookkeeper at my clinic was found to have high lipids many years ago when statins (lipid lowering drugs) had only just appeared on the Australian market. Naturally I put her on Simvastatin for trial and booked her for a repeat blood test in a few months. I was pretty convinced that all should go well and expected to see her happy and smiling on the next check-up. On the contrary, she became violently sick and started vomiting within only three days, her face had gone white and yellow, clearly due to the toxic effect of the statin. The blood test presented a picture of moderately severe upset liver functions and high bilirubin. Later on she was given a different statin (initial low dose) without the slightest upset at all! *Phew!* We learned the lesson that everyone's digestive system and immune system is different so that truly "one person's meat could be another person's poison".

Another striking example of how different chemicals will effect different individuals is a tree called the Gympie-Gympie, which is found in the northern and eastern jungles of Australia and is one of the most poisonous plants on earth. It will give anyone who simply touches its leaves extremely painful long-lasting burning sensations due to its powerful toxins that can even kill animals like dogs and horses, even though native birds, beetles and kangaroos can eat the leaves and fruit without the slightest harm!

How do we explain this? The fact is that mammals such as ourselves are extremely complex living organisms who are attuned to thrive under specific conditions which must be met for our health to be maintained. Just as a kangaroo can tolerate the Gympie-Gympie while a dog or a human cannot, we generally do not tolerate certain toxins well.

The human body is miraculous structure composed of over thirty-five trillion cells by most reasonable estimates (35,000,000, 000,000!). It is affected by all manner of factors right down to the molecular level as we shall see when we look at the research of Dr Myron Wentz, the molecular biologist, in a later section. But what happens if your body is not responding well to drug therapy and continues to deteriorate to the stage where your coronary arteries become severely blocked by cholesterol plaques? What if because of this you get chest pain while playing tennis or golf, or helping your elderly relative to lift a heavy table? Well, when things come to the worst, you will have yet a few more options of lifesaving, high-tech procedures recommended by your GP and cardiologist.

Dr Joseph Cheung

Coronary artery by-pass graft (CABG)

A Canadian surgeon Dr Arthur Vineberg (1903-1988) first implanted the mammary artery from the internal chest wall directly into the ischaemic left ventricle wall in 1960 in an operation now known as the "Vineberg procedure". It was the forerunner of modern CABG which has been greatly improved so it results in better *anastomosis* – the process of veins or arteries being joined. However, this bold yet innovative operation was quickly forgotten, and has gradually disappeared into oblivion, being replaced by a newer, much improved CABG.

CABG is a major operation consisting of cutting open the chest wall, diverting the blood into a by-pass machine which keeps the blood oxygenated and re-circulating with the heart induced into a 'sleep' mode. Then a team of surgeons will harvest healthy blood vessels and join them to the cardiovascular system of coronary arteries while by-passing the blocked area. A triple bypass utilises three new pathways while a quadruple bypass uses four. Generally veins are used as there are seldom sufficient amounts of artery to perform the procedure. Finally, the chest wall is sewed back up with steel wire to complete the operation.

The operation is probably one of the most extensive and punishing for any person, lasting from two to four hours. It's followed by a prolonged recovery which is quite painful due to the slow healing of the chest wall and ribs. So a CABG is life-saving, but not a choice you want to pick first without a serious discussion with your GP and your family. Nor would you want to repeat it.

CABG also has another problem. As veins are not as strong and durable as arteries, they may not last long, and be more easily damaged by pressure, lipid build-up and so forth. It is expensive, costing up to fifty thousand dollars US per operation. Yet in 1990 alone, three hundred and eighty thousand CABGs were carried out, despite various unpleasant complications like declining cognitive function (seventy-nine per cent), recurrent angina (chest pain) within three years, and death within ten years.

So far, nothing seems perfect. A decade after the famous by-pass procedure, a few innovative doctors started experimenting with their own ideas and a device designed to save MI patients while minimising the use of debilitating operations like CABG. First there was the European surgeon Dr Andreas Gruentzig, who conceived of introducing an inflatable balloon into the diseased coronary artery which would force open the lipid plaque-laden passage. The idea worked, and his new therapy was established and coined *angioplasty*. Having been developed further, it became a phenomenal success as far as cardiac procedures go, competing head-to-head with CABG. This has been followed by a newly designed procedure involving the use of wire springs called "stents" in place of balloons. These are coated with chemicals that discourage clotting and the build-up of lipids. Stenting is the new standard procedure which has generally replaced CABG these days because of its ease, and the fact that it delivers a fraction of the bodily punishment to the patient. The financial cost is much lower too. However, again it must be noted that nothing is perfect. Stenting itself has been found to have its own Achilles' heel – repeat stenting is common, and serious complications can arise during the procedure. Puncturing of the artery may occur, in which case the patient will require an emergency CABG.

My own attitude toward stenting is something we will go into in more detail later in the book. For now, let it suffice to say that it is not something to wade into light-heartedly, and the same for CABG and angioplasty and any other similar procedures. Because none of these expensive, high-tech, fashionable procedures are a cure for coronary artery disease (CAD). Further on we will show you more ideal ways to address CAD, which are well proven and strongly recommended by many inspiring cardiac surgeons like Prof J Kahn, Prof TC Campbell, Dr D Lundell and Dr D Ornish.

Other potholes and hazards

While CVD is the big killer, there are more minor diseases you will have to avoid if you want to be successful in your journey to longevity. In particular, you must beware of stroke (or CVA), diabetes (DM), osteoporosis and osteoarthritis (OA).

In 2003, CVA accounted for six per cent or a hundred and sixty thousand deaths in the USA; DM about three per cent or seventy-four thousand deaths. But both are set to grow to even more daunting levels of incidence in the next decades so it is vital to keep your path clear of them if you want to age healthily. Consider the following statistics.

Stroke

Every year about fifty-thousand Australians suffer a stroke, and about fifteen per cent will experience a second stroke in the first week, while twenty per cent will die within thirty days. Strokes are commonly caused either by a clot in a blood vessel in the brain (thrombotic or embolic stroke) or a rupture of the weak part in the artery (Berry's aneurysm, a congenital malformation) in a section of the brain called the Circle of Willis (haemorrhagic stroke). A common misconception is that stroke usually happens to elderly people. That is not quite true, because every year we see about two thousand people younger than forty-five in Australia also suffer a stroke, as well as another nineteen thousand who are still active in the workforce (2005 statistics).

In fact, Jill Taylor, a neuroanatomist (brain scientist), in a twist of fate, suddenly found herself struck down by an acute stroke at the young age of thirty-seven. In the end she was able to put her unique perspective on her unusual journey from wounded brain to recovery over eight years into the book *My Stroke of Insight*. The fascinating story of her experience is also recounted in the TED Talk of the same name.

How to prevent stroke? Your GP will tell you that high BP is the most important risk factor, and smoking and high lipids are the next most important things to watch out for. And if your heartbeat is irregular, you need to be properly assessed by a heart specialist and may need drugs to thin your blood. However, any blood thinning drug – called an anticoagulant – may cause a haemorrhage inside the brain too, either from a knock to the head or even as a spontaneous event. The older age group is particularly vulnerable in this regard as their blood vessel walls are weaker and less resilient; naturally, the elderly are well advised to avoid any fall and any head trauma.

Atrial fibrillation, or AF, is the most common form of irregular heartbeat. It can create clots in the fibrillating atrium (a small chamber in the left side of the heart) and you won't know when a fragment is broken off and where it will go. If it enters the brain, which is more likely than it entering the limbs or kidneys, it can temporarily upset your brain function. Such an event is termed a transient ischaemic attack (TIA), or it may simply cause a full-blown stroke which would require you to be ambulanced to hospital for immediate emergency attention.

Naturally a regular check-up of your BP is the easiest and the most important way to keep up your good health. At other times, if you experience any neurological symptoms, your GP may order a CT scan of your brain or some other tests to make sure your brain is normal anatomically and functionally. This is so an early aneurysm, if detected, could be quickly nipped off or rendered harmless by an interventional radiologist. Early treatment will save you a major brain operation and reward you with years of healthy life.

Diabetes mellitus

Many people are shocked to discover that this ailment is one of the fastest growing diseases in the civilised world. Along with hypercholesterolaemia and MI, it has been dubbed a "disease of affluence" because DM patients are commonly found in large numbers in affluent societies, feasting on rich foods, junk foods, large cans of soft drinks, and sickeningly sweet foods like cakes, sweets and rich desserts that soon overwork the pancreas with the result that it cannot produce enough insulin to handle excess sugar in the blood. Given a diet such as this, people rapidly become pre-diabetic, and then it doesn't take long for them to go down a slippery spiral to becoming a full-blown diabetic. The year 2000 revealed the terrible statistic that there were already two hundred million diabetics worldwide. That shocking number is expected to double by 2030. In fact, according to the WHO, in 2021 the figure has already more than doubled.

National surveys in many Western countries, typically the US, Britain, Australia and Canada, reveal the following common pattern: known and proven DM is found in almost four per cent of the population, plus another ten to sixteen per cent of people are pre-diabetics (based on the impaired Glucose Tolerance Test – the GTT) which adds up to about eighteen to twenty-four per cent of the total population, or roughly one in five people, being diabetic or on their way to becoming so. Pre-diabetics might experience symptoms like thirstiness, more frequent urination, increased tiredness, itchy skin, increased appetite, mildly blurred vision and some numbness in the feet or legs.

Incredibly, we are witnessing a new trend among Pacific islanders and people in many Asian countries who seem to be racing to catch up with developed countries. They are leaving behind their traditionally lower energy, low carb, high-fibre diet to feast on rich, sweet junk foods, without being taught about the many harmful consequences that arise from contracting diabetes – most disheartening.

Wake up and fight cancers

This is the last major hurdle we must overcome before we can move happily and boldly into the realm of living longer and healthier. To wage a battle effectively, you must know your enemy thoroughly. When it comes to disease, you must understand its molecular structure, the reason it arises, where it comes from, why it keeps growing bigger inside our body and spreading, and what we can do to stop it from emerging and nip it in the bud if it does.

The term *cancer* is derived from the Greek word "*karkinos*" meaning "crab" because the widespread veins and lines it causes around a breast cancer imaging (mammogram) look like the claws of a crab. There is good evidence that cancers have co-existed with humans since *Homo Sapiens* first appeared on Earth; a sort of bone cancer is said to have been found in a Javanese skeleton dating from over a million years ago.

In 2003, the US listed cancers as the number two killer, at 23 per cent of all fatalities or over half a million deaths per year. The worrying trend is that the incidence of cancers has increased thirty-seven per cent from 1950 to 1985, in the following types and order:

- Lung cancer
- Breast and colo-rectal cancer (CRC)
- Prostate cancer
- Pancreatic cancer

Now we will find out what seems to cause the above cancers. Firstly, an outstanding study regarding hereditary transmission of cancer genes was published in the NEJM in 2000. The study, which was on forty-four thousand Scandinavian identical twins, revealed that only about twenty-seven per cent of cancers are genetically linked. The rest are caused by environmental hazards like pollution and bad habits like smoking, drugs and poor diet.

Currently there are many chemicals people come into contact with or deliberately consume which are cancer-causing (carcinogenic). These include coal tar, benzopyrene from cigarette smoking, and nitrites from preserved meats such as bacon, salami and sausages. Pesticides, some of which have not been adequately tested, are another source of cancer. It may also be caused by aflatoxins, which are a family of toxins produced by certain fungi (mainly of the species aspergillus) found on certain agricultural crops like peanuts and corn. Then there are exhaust fumes from motor cars and coal-powered chimneys. Together, all these agricultural and industrial chemicals easily cause seventy to eighty per cent of all cancers. And we are not counting the fact that few people are aware of the huge number of new chemicals – roughly seventy-five thousand – that have been introduced globally in the last fifty years. With such a frightening number of new chemicals circulating in the market, it is simply impossible for the toxicologists and industrial chemists working for government public health authorities to be able to inform the public layperson which chemicals are safe, less poisonous, mildly toxic, or absolutely harmless, even to a pregnant mother and child. And this might be one of the culprits causing the ten per cent increase in childhood cancers (mainly leukaemia) over the last twenty years.

Then there is damage from radiation, including the increasingly stronger UV light from the sun due to a depleting ozone layer in the atmosphere, producing many nasty skin cancers. Australia has the highest incidence of malignant melanoma cases worldwide. We also need to watch out for radon vapour seeping out from soil and rocks as it can cause leukaemia, lymphoma and thyroid cancers. High-flyers and jet-set travellers are not immune either due to their increased exposure to cosmic rays. The list of causes is still not finished as infections from bacteria and viruses have been proven to lead to up to ten per cent of cancers. For instance, the hepatitis virus has been proven to cause liver cancer, HPV causes cervical cancer, and H pylorus in the stomach causes ulcers and cancer as well. Then there is the T-cell lymphoma virus, Burkitt's lymphoma caused by the Epstein-Barr virus, and many more!

Now it may be frightening to be confronted by so many causes of cancer, but really this is good news, because it means that this is not some mysterious curse which will strike from nowhere. You should simply consider this a list of things for you to avoid so that you don't fall prey to any of the many forms of this terrible malady.

To start with, frankly, if you stop smoking and avoid gatherings where people smoke heavily, you have already greatly reduced the chance of getting lung cancer, probably by over ninety per cent.

Additionally, as far as cancer of the breast goes, studies now point out that many of these cancers have a lot to do with being hormone-dependent, specifically on oestrogens, one of the female hormones. In other words, most breast cancers thrive well when the host's oestrogen count is high and cells are richly studded with oestrogen receptors, but will shrink and cease metastasising (spreading) if the host cell's oestrogen receptors are poor or already "coated" (meaning occupied or blocked) by a different type of oestrogen (most likely a phytoestrogen – plant sourced oestrogen, known to be a much weaker type). This is the reason why breast cancer patients take some medications – Tamoxifen for instance – which competes with cancer cells for the hormone-receptors of the host cells. This principle also appears to apply to prostate, uterine and ovarian cancers. Hence the correct treatment nowadays for such cancers is mostly immunotherapy, a simple example being the COVID-19 vaccines.

Most of my patients diagnosed with cancer of the prostate are now referred to an oncologist (cancer specialist) who will initiate a monthly injection of immunotherapy, along with strong advice to change to a plant-based diet and a healthier lifestyle. This is also regarded as an additional safeguard for some women proven to carry the oncogenes BRC 1 and 2. Of course, all of these patients need regular follow ups; for example, breast cancer cases are required to have a yearly mammogram (nowadays a 3-D type has gained more favour). And cancer prostate patients must have a blood test to track their PSA (Prostatic Specific

Antigen – a kind of enzyme secreted by the prostate gland) which generally serves as a reliable indicator of the condition of the prostate gland. Of course, keeping a check on the prostate is not complete without an annual scan, particularly if the patient complains of pain in any of their bones: the spread of cancer from the prostate to the skeletal tissue is surprisingly common.

CRC, or colo-rectal cancer, being a digestive tract cancer (a GIT), is most effectively prevented by a vegetarian diet or even one with a minimal amount of meat, as has been proven by the long-running Seventh-Day Adventist Health Study. An examination and follow-up for CRC is generally more involved as hospitalisation and repeated colonoscopy under anaesthesia is a must, in addition to scanning to see if the tumour has advanced to higher stages.

Unfortunately, pain is one of the most common symptoms in patients with cancer. Roughly about 30 to 80 per cent of patients in the early stages of the disease suffer, and between fifty to a hundred per cent at an advanced stage, according to Roger Woodruff, an Australian cancer pain specialist. At least three different types of pain, all unbearable, can occur and demand the use of a strong opioid combined with steroids, psychotropic drugs or muscle relaxants to offer the patient relief.

In 2021, a new product, Cannabi – derived from cannabis – became available from a pharmacy. It soothes anxiety and elevates the mood of people suffering from the depression generally suffered by cancer patients. Cannabis has been officially approved for cultivation at a government-run herbal farm in Tasmania for a few years, in cooperation with a Canadian set-up, to produce marijuana and hemp for medicinal therapy. The oil extract from hemp called cannabidiol is now even allowed to be infused into drinks like gin, coffee and many other new trendy beverages. This is in stark contrast to TGA (Australian government's drug agency) thinking a few years ago when all forms of cannabis were prohibited for recreational use, and anyone caught growing them would be jailed or fined. This didn't stop them from being cultivated in remote farms and in suburban homes, heavily camouflaged to avoid detection. But recent medical and therapeutic studies have found them useful for pain and mental health, provided they are taken at the correct dose and in suitable forms.

Yet, clearly, it is far better to avoid these terrible diseases than to have to find ways to deal with the pain of them. Therefore, I have provided a comprehensive section in this book on foods and diets to boost up your immune system to fight off diseases, infections and cancers, and keep you healthier and younger.

New faces of ageing

The publication in *Nature* in 2006 of Dr David Sinclair's break-through findings on genes and small molecules that can delay ageing, including the sirtuin genes, resveratrol (a plant polyphenol) and NAD precursors (Vitamin B3) made headlines all around the globe. The scientific world was stunned by Sinclair's research findings that chemicals from the plant kingdom can activate the longevity gene in laboratory animals from tiny yeast to fruit flies, worms and mice.

Not only did the animals live longer, but they were more energetic and suffered much less disease and fewer cancers. Simply put, those lab animals fed a longevity gene activator looked younger, ran more miles on a lab treadmill, had fewer grey hairs and lost more weight even when they were on high cholesterol food, in comparison to the control groups not fed the activator chemical. Autopsies provided further proof that the treated animals retained youthful organs while the untreated control group were found to have degenerated joints, heart, liver and lungs. How amazing! Thanks to twenty-five years of research, Sinclair may have finally opened up the doorway into discovering the secrets of longevity, for the first time in human history.

With ageing comes many symptoms and signs that are presented every day to GPs at clinics and hospitals in the form of CVD, cancers, diabetes, osteoarthritis, asthma and others. Medical specialists, being educated and trained in a traditional conservative fashion, which is the standard model in every medical school, usually confront such diseases and treat them in isolation and one symptom at a time. We treat and control the current disease well until the next disease erupts, and so on. Sinclair dubbed this a sort of "whack-a-mole" approach, which addresses symptoms instead of treating and irradicating the root problem and cause. This analysis seems to me to be extremely penetrating and we can expect more breakthroughs along these lines in the coming years from this brilliant researcher and his colleagues.

These perspectives are new, however, and most of us never ponder for one moment whether or not such diseases are spontaneous or due to degenerative conditions resulting from old age. Any disease in the elderly is commonly viewed as a consequence of aging; it is "bound to occur at that age", we are told that "it is just a matter of time for it to happen", or that someone is just suffering from "an old person's disease". But this common viewpoint is wrong from this new perspective. These diseases, if viewed as the symptoms and signs of ageing, require that we treat the basic cause – the ageing – long before its symptoms and signs manifest in the form as heart attacks, cancers etc., which usually start to occur during middle age, say from thirty to forty and onward.

How to treat ageing? Well, it's not as easy as treating a cancer or a flu. Just take a look at the current health strategy put up by WHO, the global medical health organisation, to combat the coronavirus. Billions have been spent on fast-tracking COVID-19 vaccine research, human trials and vaccine production, by over one hundred research centres since the start of the pandemic, and they only became available on the market at the beginning of 2021, taking most of that year to reach significant numbers of the population.

As ageing is a disease that happens to everyone – ageing is already regarded to have initiated as soon as an egg is fertilised and cells multiply in the mother's womb – so it could be viewed almost as an embryonic pandemic affecting everyone. The first thing to find out before we try to treat it are the causes that evolve into the process of ageing. Although this goes against most people's conventional thinking, it has now been accepted by increasing number of scientists and researchers. This is a good sign if more and more of the younger generation take up the challenge to push back ageing by means of the guidance we are going to mention in following chapters – simple advice like healthy lifestyles, exercise and sensible diets. It is not a constant state of illness, it is a reminder for us to keep healthy and avoid harmful habits, greed, gluttony, and other unhealthy behaviours. If this advice is followed, society will be so much better off for it.

The research to find out the answer to this question involves quite a bit of cellular, molecular, biological and genetic science. A good way to start is for us to dig deep into our cells, DNA and subcellular environment to improve our understanding, if only by a little bit. That's still better than being ignorant of what is going on with your valuable DNA inside your body and your very cells.

The incredible miracle inside your body

The exact number of cells in the human body is a matter of dispute but they are frequently estimated to be above thirty trillion. Whatever the amount, it is mind boggling and there is no doubt that each one of them is a miracle. The cell contains millions of critical molecules in the form of enzymes that are working at a frantic speed. An enzyme is about five to ten nanometres across, a nanometre being one millionth of a millimetre. It's made up of coils and layered mats of amino acid chains. One amino acid equals a single glucose molecule vibrating every quadri-millionth of a second.

The cell is an extremely busy place and its prime action is mostly concentrated in the glycolytic pathways which control glucose metabolism and the Krebs cycle, which is the final step in the oxidation of carbs, lipids and proteins. This results in the production of (ATP) adenosine, which supplies the energy, or power, for our bodies. This twenty-four-hour, non-stop process ensures that you have a continuous supply of energy to use, and indeed you are using energy every second to keep your heart pumping, lungs breathing, brain thinking, guts working. Incredible!

Every second, one of the body's enzymes – glucokinase – captures thousands of glucose molecules to be tagged on phosphorus, providing energy for RNA and ribosome to capture amino acids which will be fused to form proteins – the building blocks of our body. Each cell needs to produce over twenty thousand different proteins regularly, sourcing the correct amount and material and directing it to the right place. The break-neck speed of intracellular reaction can be illustrated by another enzyme called catalase, a detoxifying expert, which can break apart 10,000 molecules of H_2O_2 or hydrogen peroxide (toxic to the body) per second. Yet catalase is so small that a million can fit inside E. coli – the most common bacteria in our gut. And each cell has a total of seventy-five thousand enzymes like catalase.

Molecular events are incredibly fast and violent, almost mind-boggling, with molecules thrown together at speeds of possibly 1609 kilometres per hour, over and over again, up to thousands of times per second. All these subcellular events, happening every second at lightning speed, are probably beyond most readers' imagination, including mine. But why do our cells have to operate in such a big rush? A good question. Let's take a look at the incredible work all those trillions of cells have to perform day and night while we are working, yawning, eating, playing or sound asleep.

Your cells are constantly remodelling themselves while busy metabolising glucose, lipids and proteins which will be modified and sent to the cell membrane for repair, renewal and replacement of the membrane, while recycling much of the old part. The glucose so captured will serve as fuel to produce energy in the form of ATP through the famous Krebs cycle, and any left over will be modified into glycogen and stored, usually in the liver, as a future source of energy. Don't forget that each cell has to copy its own DNA in the nucleus and divide into two cells; because your body is growing, every cell needs repair, renewal and extra proteins and lipids to do the job. Thousands or even millions of cells can die if you bruise your hand or cut your skin or injure yourself in any manner, and they have to be regularly replaced anew too. About seven per cent of the body's proteins are replaced daily, and most molecules in the body are replaced every two weeks – quite an impressive rate of production and assembly of proteins and lipids. But the rate of turnover varies depending on the type of cells. For example, red blood cells last only about three weeks before requiring recycling.

Amazingly, the cells of the intestinal epithelium (the inside lining of the intestine) are being shed and replaced continuously, to the tune of seventeen billion cells daily – just imagine, seventeen billion new cells being produced while an equal number are being shed or recycled simultaneously. This mean the entire surface of the intestine is renewed every five days! Somehow your body knows it is a vitally important job to have a healthy and efficient GI tract to digest and absorb essential nutrients and vitamins so that it can supply every cell with raw material such as glucose. This generates ATP critical for energy which is used to trap all the essential amino acids required to manufacture over twenty thousand different proteins on demand, at any time. Without the intense energy produced rapidly as

ATP, the cells will cease functioning and die within minutes, even seconds. That is how critical it is to maintain a healthy gut by keeping up supplies of nutrients to every cell, organ and system of the body.

What about the biggest organ in the body, our skin? As everyone knows, skin cells are shed all the time and the amount has been estimated at three quarters of a kilo per year. Not much? But by the time you are seventy years old, you will have shed forty-eight kilos of skin cells, nearly catching up with your bodyweight! Still, we humans are fortunate compared with snakes which need to shed their entire skin after hibernation! Another of the wonders of Mother Nature.

And the skeletal system – your bones are not a static rigid scaffold either. Basically, our skeleton is just a framework of protein reinforced with calcium which forms a harder structure. It is remodelling itself continuously to respond to the feedback from your daily activities, or inactivity. The protein structure has to keep changing its shape and angle in response to gravitational pull, and to the direction of muscular forces every minute during your movements and exercises. Calcium minerals are constantly removed and built up by osteoclasts and osteoblasts, bone cells of opposing function. Osteoclasts act to dissolve the bone, while osteoblasts build up bone, influenced and controlled by the parathyroid hormones which become most active during puberty so you grow taller each year.

With that much heavy work repairing, replacing and reproducing every part of your body every minute and every second, isn't it a miracle that we are still alive, even for thirty seconds? We ought to remind ourselves that our body, unlike a simple one-cell organism such as a yeast cell or even a bacterium like E. coli, is a highly advanced, multi-organ unit, with a highly developed central nervous system, protective immune system and creative brain. We cannot afford to have any part of our body missing or not functioning properly, nor can we allow any interruption to our naturally intense cellular metabolism. It is all of this which makes us Homo sapiens, and what Sinclair proclaimed us to be, great survivors.

The cell nucleus remains the supreme controller of all intra-cellular activities with its DNA, the double-helix formation of molecules which contains all of the information for the cell to function. This is despite the fact that it has long been known that nearly eighty per cent of it is inactive: what is referred to as "junk DNA". The functioning of our bodies, therefore, relies on the remaining twenty per cent, or thirty thousand genes, to organise amino acids to form some twenty thousand different types of protein. It is somewhat intriguing to consider that the cells in your body are somehow communicating with each other using a delicate feedback network which controls the type and the amount of proteins, lipids and glucose required, every minute of your life.

DNA is tightly packed inside the cell nucleus. If you are curious and have the skill to pick out the DNA molecule in a cell and stretch it out, it could reach a length of two metres. By extension it has been calculated that, if all the DNA in your body (one hundred trillion of them) were stretched out and connected together, the line would reach to the moon and back! Again, a truly mind-boggling concept.

Apart from being damaged in obvious ways by exposure to X rays, radiation, chemicals, toxins or cigarette smoke, DNA is also damaged in the normal process of copying/replication in a cell's growth cycle. Therefore, cells rely heavily on enzymes (up to a hundred or more) to repair damaged or broken strands for the cell to survive and return to normal.

The mitochondria are your body's factory at the subcellular level, or the powerhouse where nutrients are broken down to create energy. As your body cannot afford to have energy production interrupted even for one second, just as a factory cannot afford to have its power supply cut off because it will cause an instant blackout and the breakdown of the machinery of production, this cellular component is regarded as one of the chief indicators of ageing. The power and energy comes from the ATP produced from the Krebs cycle in the metabolism of glucose, as mentioned earlier. So it may not surprise you to learn that mitochondria are most highly concentrated in the most active body parts or organs, like muscle cells, which can contain up to two thousand mitochondria ready to generate up to one billion ATP molecules to provide energy during strenuous sport activities such as a running a marathon or playing in a rugby match.

The cell membrane is what the nucleus uses to protect the chromosome and DNA, but allows certain enzymes and molecules in and out to facilitate repair, replication and communication. Naturally, a cell also needs a special wrapping – a sort of "fluid mosaic" composed of lipids and proteins that is selectively permeable by small molecules, RNA messengers etc., with an added facility for using ATP to actively transport nutrients in and expel wastes. But take note that the membrane itself is also replaced and modified constantly and rapidly as the lipid molecules last only hours and the protein component may wear out in days.

Ageing

Now that we have discovered the structure and components of a cell, and its working modes, it is a little bit easier for us to look under the inscrutable mask of ageing to figure out what the process really entails.

Since the human desire to live longer has always been fascinating to most people, there have been many interesting theories and proposals since the 1930s when scientists at Cornell University found out that rodents on starvation or calorie restriction (CR) diets lived longer. We have also explored some of the theories such as "DNA damage" and "DNA copying mistakes" which cause gene mutation, and the popular theory of "oxidative stress and damage" to DNA and mitochondria being a powerful cause of ageing. It is true that mitochondria decline is one of the hallmarks of ageing, but it may be that ageing could be treated and reversed easily.

Nevertheless, none of the theories and proposals have stood the test of time. Only the "oxidative damage and stress" concept still remains attractive, notably backed up with enthusiasm by pharmaceutical and nutraceutical manufacturers – it is still a five billion dollar industry, with hundreds of "anti-oxidant" products on offer including ointments, pills and powders which boast of rapid relief of oxidative stress; the "scientifically proven" enhancement of the protective power of your immune system, and "reliable supplements" to fend off many illnesses and maintain your youth. In reality, hundreds of scientific studies and experiments have been carried out without any clear-cut proof that antioxidants help lab animals live significantly longer.

The cause of ageing, as discussed before, is a loss of information in the cells – the information that tells you who you are and how you live and grow and survive.

There are two kinds of information – the first type is the *digital,* as encoded in the three billion base pairs (four nucleotide base pairs in special sequence) in our DNA. Although it is commonly believed that nearly eighty per cent of our DNA genome has been found to be "junk" or not considered useful, the remaining twenty per cent was nearly completely mapped in 2003, or as much as it could be given the technology of the time. That was a mammoth project involving hundreds of scientists in many countries, lasting over ten years and at a cost of one billion dollars. Each of the three billion pairs of genes making up the human genome was identified. DNA is robust and so the genetic information can be copied hundreds of times and passed on to generation after generation; in other words, the information is hereditary, and capable of being transmitted by genetic means. It is like computer memory stored digitally on a hard disc, and can be retrieved intact numerous times.

The second kind of information is *analogue*, which is now more commonly known as "epigenome" and stored in chromatin or strands of DNA as traits, heritable but not transmitted by genetic means. Genetically, this is like the software on your computer – it orchestrates a fertilised cell to develop into a newborn with trillions of cells and specialised organs and tissue. It dictates and controls all the functions of the cell and every organ. Simply put, it is the supreme commander of your whole body. It is versatile and capable of meeting new challenges by switching genes on and off for the survival of the organism or animal.

Genes can be switched on and off by SIRT1 (sirtuin 1) – the longevity gene discovered by D Sinclair – by taking off or adding chemical tags, commonly methyl and acetyl radicals, without affecting the four base pairs of nucleotides of DNA (there are three billion base pairs on the DNA).

The major disadvantage of this epigenomic information, however, being analogue, is that it is not as robust and stable as the digital information, and can be lost while being copied, or when being X-rayed, or when invaded by viruses, or by external chemicals and toxins, notably toxic chemicals from cigarettes.

Starting from when the earth was formed four billion years ago, our primitive ancestor – nicknamed *Magna superstes* by David Sinclair (meaning "great survivor" in Latin) had somehow evolved with a competitive edge due to an extra function of its genes, which were capable of repairing damaged and broken DNA so the organism could survive in a harsh relentless environment, much to the blessing of all its descendants today carrying out this survival circuit in a more or less similar form – mammals, fish, birds, trees, insects and all other living things.

The primordial life form of *Magna superstes* had two genes for the survival circuit, but mammals are now found to have two dozen or more of these in our genome, which scientists fondly refer to as "longevity genes" or "vitality genes" because they help us to live longer, protect us against diseases and infections, and help us to remain endowed with energy and so stay healthier. These genes form a complicated surveillance network by means of special proteins and chemicals, supplied via the blood stream, which communicate with each other and exercise control over our body.

The longevity genes

In his pursuit to discover the contributors to a long life span, David Sinclair has chosen the clever strategy of studying tiny yeast cells as their life-cycle is short, only about twenty-one days, or twenty-five divisions, so that the effects of chemicals etc., for better or for worse, can be observed, measured and recorded within a month or two. This has the huge advantage of allowing many observations to be made over a short period of time.

Within a few years working in his lab at Harvard Medical School, he found the molecule that could activate the longevity gene so the yeast cell lived fifty per cent longer. Subsequent experiments have indicated equally exciting effects on worms, fruit flies and rodents. Trials with humans in 2018 suggested that the survival circuit has not changed significantly after four billion years of turbulent events on this earth. The molecule he has discovered is sirtuin, named after the yeast Sir2 gene. Sirtuins are enzymes descended from the clever gene in *Magna superstes* or whatever other primordial organism existed at the time.

SIRTS are made by almost every cell in our body: there are seven in mammals, which have been found to specialise at performing different tasks. SIRT 1, 6, and 7 exercise control of epigenome and DNA repair. SIRT 3, 4 and 5 reside inside mitochondria and control energy production. SIRT 2 is required to supervise cellular division and healthy egg production. So these sirtuins are epigenetic regulators and work by attaching or removing chemical groups like acetyl and methyl tags, changing DNA packaging and turning genes on and off. They act as the commander and controller of all DNA repair, all reproduction, fitness, health and of course survival.

Another chemical Sinclair has discovered is TOR (or Target of Rapamycin) which, similar to sirtuins, is found in every cell, performing similar functions: DNA repair, control of inflammation, improvement of survival, and a special function designed to digest old and unwanted proteins.

All the above information on genetics, although rather technical, is intended to help the readers comprehend better the core of longevity which is an unavoidably complex science involving many fields, including basic biology, medicine and genetics, as well as knowledge of the mechanisms operating at the subcellular level of our body.

I hope it will have impressed upon the reader what a walking miracle their body is. How tragic it would be to squander such an incredible work of evolution by subjecting it to such unnecessary and avoidable stresses as those which lead to cancer and heart attack, which I have described the dangers of already. When we see how hard our body is working every day, performing all of these miracles in every single cell, hopefully we will be inspired to help it in its never-ending efforts to keep us energised, stable and healthy, rather than undermining its efforts.

In the following chapters we will explore more fully the many paths that lead to a healthier and more enjoyable longevity and strike out into some exciting new territory as well.

Chapter Five: Let's Push Back Ageing

In human history, it appears that our ancestors were already curious about the biology of birth, living, and death, as is vividly shown by an exchange, recorded over twenty-five thousand years ago, between a student and Confucius, the famed Chinese sage. Confucius, or *Kong Fu Zi* in Chinese – literally "Master Kong" – was born in 551 BC, during the Warring Kingdoms period. He continuously toured all seven kingdoms with his students, teaching and lecturing and enlightening the kings, court ministers and the general public who were enthralled by his moral philosophy.

Confucius died in 479 BC, but his moral teachings and profound philosophy have had an enormous influence on the Chinese, generation after generation, and continue to do so even today. His ideas and advice were recorded by his teams of disciples, in printed form, and have been used by scholars throughout the greater part of Chinese history up to the modern era where they are taught in high school as well as university. His teachings, based on a specific code of appropriate personal and national moral values and behaviour can be viewed as the bible for all Chinese, individuals and governments alike.

In a particular teaching session, according to the record, one of his brightest students named Kwai Lo put this question to Confucius: "Master, why do young people keep growing up, to become old and die? What has made them age and die? And what is it like after death?" To this difficult enquiry in a time without the benefit of modern scientific knowledge the great philosopher replied, "you see a woman giving birth and the baby starting to grow? We don't even know how and why the baby is born and gifted with life, so how can we understand how and why a living man ages and dies?"

So the best the greatest mind of his day could really do, two and a half thousand years ago, was to deflect the question by reflecting upon the general state of ignorance of humanity. It is a strikingly different story today. Why? Well, as we have seen, from years of demographic surveys and studies on the longest lived humans in the Blue Zones both in the East (Bapan in China, Okinawa near Japan) and the West (Sardinia in Italy, Loma Linda in California), it is fairly clear that a significant number of people can live into their nineties, hundreds and even to as old as a hundred and ten and over – the super-centenarians. But, as pointed out in Chapter Three, there are many dominant features in the Blue Zones and the centenarians' lifestyle that are different to those of us living elsewhere, and we may never be able to emulate or fit these into our lives.

But do not despair; take heart. Looking beyond the chaos of the coronavirus, it is nonetheless clear that under normal circumstances most people, particularly in the thirty- to fifty-year-old group when the disease of ageing starts calling, can do a lot to delay the inevitable. In this chapter, I will show you all the different ways to push back ageing, to prevent devastating diseases including cancers, to give you a healthier body and a longer and healthier life to enjoy with your family. This is now becoming more and more a reality and a dream come true, all due to centuries of study, hard work and perseverance by brilliant scientists and researchers with inquiring minds, culminating in the latest breakthrough discovery by David Sinclair that some chemicals and enzymes can activate our longevity gene and bypass the awkward old method of caloric restriction, which although reliable is difficult to perform in practice.

The followings methods are for anyone who wishes to lead a longer and healthier life. Some are well proven through lab experiments on animals and also through data gathered in the study of the Blue Zones. Others are newly discovered chemicals, enzymes and even hi-tech inventions and genetic materials that may need more evaluation in future.

Caloric restriction (CR)

CR is a well proven way to achieve a longer life that dates back to centuries ago. It was first proven in the lab with experiments on rodents in 1930 at Cornell University, when rats fed forty per cent less were observed to live fifty per cent longer. CR has since been proven to be beneficial for all life forms, including rhesus monkeys which were the focus of a study begun in 1980.

In the Blue Zone of Bapan village in southwest China near Vietnam, the villagers usually get up early and commence their farm work without breakfast, working until night-time before returning home to have dinner with the family – which means almost sixteen hours of fasting during the day. This habit seems to give the system a chance to optimize and reset the hormone IGF-1 (insulin growth factor-1). Since the word spread about Bapan, the village has become a mecca for longevity enthusiasts, attracting a steady stream of people from many parts of China wishing to learn how to extend their life spans.

Okinawans appear to carry out similar CR even though they don't skip breakfast. When they sat down for meals with the investigating scientists, they insisted on eating until they were only about eighty per cent full. Compared with the Japanese on the mainland, Okinawans take in twenty per cent fewer calories, thereby maintaining a fit, lean body with a BMI (Body Mass Index) of within eighteen to twenty, a very healthy body weight by any standard (in everyday medical practice, the standard BMI is considered to be between twenty and twenty-five).

If such fulltime regular practice of CR is not your cup of tea (and it is something few people relish), then try a modified form called "intermittent" or "periodic" fasting, which is almost like what is practised daily in Bapan. That may also lower your IGF-1. Simply put, hunger turns on genes in the brain that release longevity hormones.

So CR success has been well proven in animals, from yeast to rodents, but has never had a clear-cut benefit shown in experiments on human volunteers. This is because, firstly, the time frame necessary to show unequivocal benefits in life span has to be a reasonably long one in order to deliver significant improvements, say at least a few months and even up to a few years. During this time, the subjects would have to be confined to a camp or a building, and have to be checked, and supervised, at all times to prevent cheating on food rations if they become unable to stand semi-starvation and start desperately looking for tasty pizzas or take-away food, or in case they fall ill for some reason, the most probable one being depression and anxiety due to confinement and boredom.

The situation could be comparable to the hotel quarantine imposed on overseas travellers returning to Australia in Melbourne during the COVID-19 pandemic in 2020. Untrained "guards" were employed instead of police or military personnel, and they had no idea how to carry out the rules, nor to maintain discipline themselves. News and rumours abounded with media images of some of the night guards who just slept on the floor outside the room being guarded, so soundly at times that some, perhaps many, coronavirus-infected guests had no trouble slipping in and out of their rooms at will, spreading the virus and causing the explosive second wave in Melbourne. Some "guards" also tested positive after being "too friendly" with infected guests. Naturally this mismanagement turned into a media scandal and ended up being under inquiry, Royal Commission style.

The result? Not a single person, from the premier to the lowest ranking officials, admitted making a wrong decision. Eventually no one was found guilty, and the chaos with other mishaps and mismanagement seems to have been white-washed after the lockdown relaxed in October of that year. Clearly experiments on humans are never an easy task and not to be attempted lightly, particularly on a long-term basis.

Exercise for vitality

If you don't feel like practising CR and consider it a kind of torture, gastronomically speaking, you may well welcome exercise as an alternative.

Throughout the history of medicine, exercise has been quoted as the most beneficial thing you can easily do for your body and mind. In fact, the great Greek physician Hippocrates, often referred to as the "Father of Medicine" and the founder of the Hippocratic School of Medicine way back about two thousand four hundred years ago, was already promoting exercise as evidenced by his maxim that "walking is man's best medicine".

Then, four hundred years ago, the English physician William Harvey demonstrated the human circulatory system through anatomical teaching (autopsy), and doctors were able to visualise the connection between exercise and good circulation of the blood supplying every organ, improving cardiovascular output, pulmonary function, and leading to stronger muscles and better health.

But doctors have not been able to explain the correlation of exercise with longevity until recently, in 2017, when a study led to the discovery of at least one of the reasons. Research conducted on the subcellular level revealed that people who exercised well were found to have longer telomeres, the end part of a chromosome which protects the integrity of the structure from damage. This significance of telomeres in regard to aging is a fairly recent discovery by subcellular biologists, who found that they were shortened every time a cell divides and chromosomes copy themselves. After a certain number of cell divisions, the telomere shortens to nothing, so the cell becomes senescent – ages – and dies. It has been thought that the telomere could be a protective mechanism designed by nature to prevent the cell from growing uncontrollably like a tumour. Afterward, scientists discovered an enzyme called telomerase which can extend the telomeres – genetically restoring youthfulness and pushing back ageing. For this work, one of the team, the Australian-American scientist Elizabeth Blackburn, shared the Nobel prize along with Carol Greider and Jack Szostak. So this knowledge that telomere shortening is one of the signs of ageing, and can be manipulated more easily with suitable chemicals and methods is something new and exciting.

Returning to the benefits of exercise: I myself have always been an advocate for exercise. My brothers and I trained at the swimming pool every summer school break. This was the only time we could possibly spare because study and passing exams had to be our overriding priority in the very competitive environment of Hong Kong in the years after WWII. We managed to collect a few trophies and prizes to show off and please our father, who was himself a champion rower in his university days, and regularly spurred us on to keep training in sports.

Much to my regret, that idyllic time had to end as I commenced my studies at the University of Sydney, and I did not really resume my sporting activities until well after my return to Melbourne and entry into general practice. And everyone knows what general practice is like: face-to-face consultation, a lot of talking to heavy-breathing, coughing patients carrying all sorts of viruses who were not always mindful of common-sense hygiene. Within a few years, and with recurrent colds, sore throats and sinus infections, I could feel that my immune system was deteriorating most notably in the winter months in Melbourne. There I experienced its famous "four seasons in one day"; a bright sunny morning that rapidly transformed into a cold windy late morning which might even be followed by snow falling in the outer suburbs! Such changeability is obviously rather dramatic to tourists and non-Melbournians.

Subconsciously, I knew I had to do something to enhance my body's resistance to viruses and bacteria, and that I could not rely on the legacy of fitness and good health from my younger days lasting forever. So I forced myself back into the swimming pool and supplemented that activity with jogging. And, you know what, for the next thirty-five years at the same clinic, I have not had to take a single day off sick! I even worked longer hours to handle an increasing number of patients as the longest-serving senior partner, while one of the youngest partners never stopped complaining of his "heavy" workload until he left the clinic after a few years.

That was the turning point in my thinking, when I began to see the benefits of regular exercise. It had clearly strengthened my immune system, protected me against all sorts of common ailments like flus and colds, conferred more energy upon me and generally given me better health. There is no greater proof than one's own experience. I soon discovered that few of my patients exercised and I saw quite a few fall victim to MI, asthma or diabetes. In North America, it has been reported that less than five per cent of people do regular exercise. Worse still, in China, even children are now doing fifty per cent less exercise compared with their parents a generation ago.

The end result? With less exercise and more junk food, the situation has already deteriorated into a global health crisis dominated by overweight and obesity, which brings with it all the diseases of affluence, notably CVD, HBP, NIDDM and OA. Obviously, this also impacts anyone's chances of ageing well and enjoying a long life.

When I first began my exercise programme, although I never correlated exercise with the benefit of living longer, I already had an intuition that my regular training would not only protect me from seasonal viral infections, but also that it could contribute to me enjoying a longer life. I often found myself quietly reflecting on my family history. My father and two older brothers all succumbed to cancers and died roughly at the age of eighty. I, on the other hand, am now eighty-six, and I have just retired, albeit reluctantly, after fifty-nine years working hard as a GP. Some heart trouble was discovered over ten years ago which showed up on a CT coronary angiogram (CTCA) in the form of an almost completely blocked main artery, but functionally my heart seems happy to keep going with the help of quite a few collateral arteries compensating. My interventional cardiologist Dr G Lau considered stenting not advisable due to the heavily calcified narrow entrance (the ostia), meaning stenting or other operative procedures might not be effective, or even cause further complications with my heart. My other systems are still quite sound and I reckon, if not for the pandemic, I could have kept working for a few more years, maybe even to ninety or beyond.

My conclusion was that I had to decide to rely on non-operative ways to improve my heart. Yet my constitution as a child was never as strong as that of my older brother, who was Sydney University's basketball team captain during his days there studying dentistry. He was always fit and "strong as a Mallee bull", to borrow a phrase one of my regular patients would always use when I enquired about his health.

So I have my own sneaking suspicions that all my health, stamina, endurance, and extended life, could be attributed to my years of regular physical training. There's nothing pie in the sky about that, particularly now that exercise has been discovered to be one of the strong positive stressors (we will list more stressors later) in our lives which serve to activate all the known longevity regulators and all our survival circuit networks – these include the sirtuins AMPK and mTOR, all modulated to the right direction, and SIRT 1 and SIRT 6, which can help extend telomeres and package them up to prevent fraying, resulting in a more durable Telomere to facilitate pushing back ageing – one of the key pieces of the longevity jigsaw.

Technically, exercise is usually divided into anaerobic and aerobic modes, with the latter being the most popular and considered the healthiest type to follow, which is why that is what I am referring to specifically by the term "exercise" in this book. It will benefit your body in numerous ways.

The effects of exercise kicks in about fifteen minutes after you commence it. When you are jogging, running, swimming or cycling, for example, your large muscle groups burn off the fatty acid in the fatty tissue by utilising the oxygen you breath in and producing energy, water and carbon dioxide. The latter two are quickly and easily expelled as simple waste. Meanwhile, glycogen is also metabolised into ATP energy. The amount of glucose in the blood during moderately strenuous exercise has been reported to be up to four hundred times higher than while in a sedentary state. This means that by exercising you lose fatty tissue and lower your blood sugar at the same time. In a report published in *The Guardian*, from a study by Harvard Medical School in 1990, seventy-five per cent of doctors surveyed were found to exercise regularly, and diet on top of that. Many of them were expected to live to ninety or close to it if they stuck to their healthy lifestyles.

Your muscles are the biggest consumer of your daily calorie intake, estimated to use up to ninety per cent of your daily energy output. They become bigger from regular exercise and continuously but quietly burn up more and more of your body fat – what a blessing from above for those who are overweight.

The heart is one of the organs receiving a huge benefit from exercise which will develop a stronger, better-tuned myocardium (heart muscle), open up more collaterals (side branches from the coronary arteries) and help supply more blood to the cardiac muscles. It can help bypass partly blocked arteries and may spare you an expensive angioplasty (a procedure to open up blocked arteries, costing over thirty thousand dollars, US) or an equally expensive stenting procedure, or even a much more expensive CABG (bypass surgery, up to fifty thousand dollars) if the other procedures fail or are too difficult.

Not less important are the cholesterol-lowering effects from exercise – there will be a reduction of LDL, the bad cholesterol, and a simultaneous elevation of HDL, the good cholesterol. The HDL is believed to act like a scavenger which controls the build-up of LDL, by secreting an enzyme to protect the arterial wall. It has been discovered by D. Lundell, a cardiac procedurist, that eighty per cent of heart attacks come from burst LDL soft plaque in the coronary artery and less frequently from a thrombotic event. The LDL plaque can become soft due to oxidative damage and a lack of the HDL's protective mechanism.

This theory fits in quite well with my experience working on three hundred or more autopsies during my three years in the pathology department in the combined Ottawa General and Civic Hospitals of Canada. Most of the time, only a small percentage of coronary arteries were found to have a clear-cut thrombus, even though (usually) large and extensive calcified plaques are unmistakably dotted all along the major branches. Although the precise mode of action of HDL and that of LDL are as yet to be unravelled through further research, the linear relationship between high total cholesterol (LDL) and a high rate of MI is beyond dispute.

Hypercholesterol condition is very common in Australia, as it is in most countries where a diet high in land-animal meat and dairy is standard. According to professor Tonkins of the National Heart Foundation, it was found in from forty to fifty per cent of the population as estimated in surveys conducted from 1980 to 2000. Yet surprisingly, the American Heart Association's yearly statistics in 2013 estimated that only thirteen per cent of Americans were over the mark, even though over sixty per cent of them were overweight and obese. Maybe more Americans heeded the warnings after Bill Clinton's MI and quadruple bypass and began to consume more statins (cholesterol lowering pills), or such a statistical difference is due to varying standards for lab data criteria.

In his 2005 book *China Study*, Colin Campbell, Professor of Nutritional Biochemistry at Cornell University, concluded twenty years of nutritional research conducted in a partnership between Cornell, Oxford University and the Chinese Academy of Preventive Medicine. The findings showed that cholesterol levels in China were much lower: CHD (coronary heart disease) was, in fact, seventeen times lower than in North America! The rate of cancers in all major organs was also much lower. Professor Campbell was particularly startled by the extraordinarily low rate of CHD in Guizhou and Sichuan provinces, where, over the span of three years, it was found that for the subject population of half a million, *not a single case* of CHD death had been reported in a person younger than sixty-four. He pointed to their very healthy diet of plant proteins as a powerful cholesterol-lowering factor. When Campbell checked the records and statistics, he could see a striking difference: on the one hand, the Americans got eighty per cent of their protein from animal products like meat, milk, cheese and eggs. This formed more than 10 per cent of their daily calorie intake. On the other hand, rural Chinese derived less than one per cent of their calories from animal products.

So the relationship between diet, cholesterol and CHD has never been illustrated more clearly than by Campbell's comprehensive studies: the higher the animal protein in your diet, the higher the cholesterol level in your blood; the higher the cholesterol in the blood, the greater the chance of heart attack. This all seems unbelievably simple and far from exciting, but it has taken many dedicated researchers and scientists years to come up with this concrete solution to the riddle.

In 1984, researcher H.B. Simon found that exercising muscles helped increase HDL. This finding was confirmed in 2003 by Baker's Heart Research Institute in Melbourne. Another unexpected benefit from exercise was discovered in a study by a German research team. They divided post-angioplasty patients into two groups: one group was required to exercise daily while the other remained mostly sedentary. After only one month, they found the exercise group had double the rate of blood flow in their coronary arteries compared with the non-exercise group. On further testing, they concluded that the reason was the increase of nitric oxide released in their circulation during exercise. Nitric oxide works powerfully to dilate the arteries, thereby inducing increased blood flow to the heart.

That the effect and benefit of exercise does vary according to the intensity with which it engages the greater number of longevity genes, is a finding that was also confirmed by a new study on 2000 men in Wales reported by the British Heart Foundation. The research demonstrated that vigorous activities such as swimming, jogging and climbing stairs confers maximum protection to the heart and elevates physical fitness to the highest degree. While not as effective, moderate exercise such as that afforded by digging, dancing and golfing is still beneficial. However, little benefit is gained from just leisurely walking and bowling. There are also indications that exercise induces the mitochondria to burn off more oxygen and generate more energy, which again indirectly helps the immune system.

In addition to all of the above benefits, regular exercise provides other fringe benefits such as a slower heart rate which cuts down that vital organ's workload. It increases your BMR, which in turn improves circulation and immune response, and stimulates the production of the much talked about endorphins and enkephalins in the brain, which give athletes that high that has them feeling on top of the world.

Cold and sauna exposure

The idea that these two stimuli can be used to help push back ageing is something new and will seem unusual to many readers. According to Professor David Sinclair, a regular cold dip will turn on your longevity genes by producing more "brown fat" in your body. Brown fat is abundant in babies and children but disappears fast as one grows older. The point is that brown fat is mitochondria rich and provides you with more energy and vitality.

Obviously, jumping into cold or icy cold water will shock anyone not used to it. It may not be everybody's cup of tea, and only when you try it will you get an idea of how easy it will be for you to develop this habit, if you choose to take advantage of its benefits. For myself, after three years in the freezing climate in Ottawa, even a romantic image of riding along and singing "Jingle Bells" with Santa Claus on his reindeer sleigh is not enough to tempt me. The comfort of Sydney's mild weather has much more alure in my case.

The famed northern European sauna, so popular with the locals, is said to be another stimulus for the immune system which relies on heat, as opposed to cold. It can be quite hot and dry and to some simply feels like being roasted. There aren't that many good solid studies on the benefits to present a particularly convincing case so is up to the user to try it out.

A healthy lifestyle

Before WWII, people hardly worried about their "style" of life. After 1918, with the end of WWI, many nations were busy re-building their infrastructure, re-establishing trade, commerce, education and food supplies. However, WWII was even more devastating, with the world suffering under the aggression of Germany, Italy and Japan, who had banded together with an insane dream to conquer the whole planet: Germany and Italy would swallow Europe, Britain and Russia while the Japan would occupy all of China and Southeast Asia. This led to their infamous sneak attack on the USA's main naval base at Pearl Harbour. Even Darwin in Australia's Northern Territory did not escape unscathed.

Because the aggressors were well prepared, with their huge arsenal of advanced weapons and their armies were so well trained, the scope and intensity of the war was something the world had never seen before. Lives were destroyed in their millions by the increasingly advanced and destructive firepower used on land and at sea, while bombs rained from the skies.

Our family home in Japanese-occupied Hong Kong missed a direct hit from the allied bombers in one of their night attacks – the huge bomb landed on a peddler's shed next to our neighbour's building with such powerful force and deafening noise that our younger sister jumped out of her bed and came flying into our bedroom screaming for help. That's war, and bombs can fall anywhere. As I search my soul in retrospect, I see that we were exceptionally lucky: we suffered no injury, our house remained intact, and none of us were killed. It was just a close shave and a war-time episode never to be forgotten. But in time you come to realise many thousands of people have had similar or even more frightening experiences they never narrate.

The war ended in 1945. The aggressors were soundly defeated and duly disgraced as they surrendered to the Allies to face severe punishment. The would-be conquerors became the conquered, and a badly traumatised world slowly and painfully picked itself up again, beginning where it had left off after WWI. Millions of people were killed and maimed in WWII, the majority of them mostly from innocent and peace-loving families. The legacy of that terrible period of history is a mountain of the most heartbreaking images of hardship and suffering experienced globally, for which those aggressive criminal governments can never repay nor compensate.

But what has all this got to do with lifestyle? Well, if you recall that baby boomers in Australia are those born after the war (1946-1965). This boomer generation, in developed countries, has apparently been well-cared for throughout and enjoyed world-class education and university studies. When they completed their tertiary education and began searching for jobs, it was like a dream compared to what youngsters today must face because the unemployment rate in that era was, at times, below one per cent!

But in all the developed nations, people have more or less changed their lifestyles dramatically, copying their American cousins, campaigning for freer sex, or experimenting with addictive drugs like marijuana or amphetamines. They have enjoyed social status, they have money and good earning power. They occupy important government positions and are active in every respectable profession, businesses and research institution. They take regular holidays at the seaside; they're sun-tanned and inclined to indulge in long lunches with an unlimited supply of grog.

Therefore, it seems by all indications that the baby boomers have been having a good time and enjoying their lifestyles. But they cannot be said to be healthy ones, or to engender a long lifespan. As you will see, from the '70s onward, many of the boomers noticed that something was going awry. They started to suffer CVD and increasing incidents of heart attack, even when as young as thirty-five or forty. And in those days, the majority of emergency patients I and many other young doctors rostered on in "Casualty" (it was not yet named "Emergency") saw in the early morning or late at night – the most common times of day for heart trouble – presented with acute chest pain and were found to have suffered a classic attack heart. In that era, without hi-tech procedures, some patients' lives could be saved in the Intensive Care Unit, but many just succumbed to a massive heart attack. There were no miracle drugs for heart attack and no surgeons dared to put a tube into the coronary artery to probe around.

CVD and MI are bad enough and frightening, but the trouble does not stop there. Many other diseases surfaced soon after to attack the boomers, such as diabetes, asthma, stroke, lung cancers, breast cancers, obesity, osteoarthritis and bowl cancers. Anyone who has the misfortune of suffering any of these chronic and frequently fatal illnesses often also develops mental illness like anxiety or depression, which may even lead to suicide. Talking about the latter, I can assure you that it is not uncommon for desperate patients to take the road of self-destruction to escape their ills. Just in my time working in the largest charity hospital in Hong Kong, I personally witnessed a few patients climb over barriers in the ward and jump to the ground from the fifth or sixth floor! It is quite a shocking experience for anyone to see a suicide like that. The victims are often the chronically ill, who after suffering severe pain for a long time, see no hope of getting well and become filled with despair.

What does all this mean? Just that by simply acknowledging all the advantages of baby boomers' lives does not necessarily indicate that they are truly happy. Many of them do not have the disease-free, healthy life that you and I are seeking. I am particularly interested in advising my readers to follow a healthy lifestyle as below, in order to achieve not just a longer lifespan, but real healthy ageing: disease-free, cancer-free, pain-free, a longer, more energetic life full of joy and purpose.

Exercise
Probably the most important contributor to a healthy lifestyle; ample evidence has already been given for this above.

Avoiding smoking
Many years ago, Australian actor and film icon Paul Hogan – "Crocodile Dundee" – often appeared on TV ads promoting smoking, in the most relaxed and casual manner, by charming the audience with his catch phrase "Have a Winfield"! A very

simple ad but surprisingly effective, literally enticing thousands of teens like magic to copy his style and start smoking this brand of cigarette. It might even have been a subtle factor later on in the rising tide of young girls picking up smoking leading to the unfortunate, sharply increasing rate of lung cancer and death in females trying to catch up with males in recent years.

If someone asks you what kills the most people on earth, what would your answer be? Motor car accidents? An influenza epidemic? Heart disease? The great wars of WWI or WWII? Or the recent Covid-19 pandemic? Well, none of those! The biggest of all the mega killers is actually smoking tobacco! According to the figure announced during World No Tobacco Day (31 May 2004) by the WHO, five million smokers die every year from tobacco-related illnesses. Not just in one particular year, but every year, and the figure seems to be rising and is expected to reach 10 million by 2025. Is this a new trend or just ignorance and the addictive power of nicotine, with the world's tobacco companies, like drug cartels, as the prime movers?

Cigarettes are not getting cheaper either, the price keeps rising ever higher due to the steeply increasing taxes imposed by governments all over the world in an all-out effort to "butt out" smoking to protect people's lives. Studies have found that a life will be cut short by seven minutes for every cigarette, and smoking has been implicated as a possible cause of chest pain (angina) as spasms of the coronary artery have been observed while a person was smoking in an angiogram photo published by a reputable medical journal (the New England Journal of Medicine).

A passive smoker who inadvertently consumes second-hand smoke – the smoke created by smokers – might get away with a less harsh penalty to their health, but you must try your best to avoid ingesting this poison, given that, as the US Surgeon-General warned, twenty years of scientific research has shown that there is no safe level of passive smoking, and there is no absolute proof that any currently employed air-filtration device can get rid of cigarette smoke and its health hazards. Tobacco leaves contain several thousand types of chemicals (WHO July 2021), and of these, at least 250 of them are harmful, many being carcinogens, so tobacco is inherently addictive as well as being a multi-poison, even in minute amounts. WHO has declared all forms of tobacco are harmful and there is no safe level of exposure. The carcinogens can damage your DNA, causing breakage. We are not sure how many breaks happen, but it may be dependent on how many packets a day you smoke, and how you inhale, as well as other factors like how many years you have been smoking.

Every time DNA break, sirtuin genes rush to the damage sites to initiate repairs and protect the cell. This may easily be done initially, but as the smoking causes more damage and DNA breakage, the exhausted sirtuins may not be able to cope that well and may even lose their way home. So, slowly your vitality genes become run down and weaker, and they cannot stop mutations in some of the lining cells of the bronchial trees, leading to the next step of malignant change. As the process advances further, the smoker starts to present with the first symptoms of haemoptysis (coughing up blood), undue shortness of breath, or unexplained chest infections which commonly present as partial pneumonia. By this stage it can be too late and the smoker can require specialist therapy. Unfortunately, the mortality rate from lung cancer is very high: only one in seven sufferers is saved. Even then, life after a lung cancer operation will never be the same as usually a carer is required, and often a portable oxygen tank will have to tag along anywhere the victim goes – what a miserable lifestyle!

Smoking is a great waste of money. Just a few years ago in Australia, the market research company AC Nelson revealed research showing that Australians burnt up four to five billion dollars' worth of cigarettes, just from supermarkets alone. Isn't it ridiculous that it is often the ordinary workers who can least afford to spend money on unnecessary items that choose to smoke, while many intelligent and educated persons usually act the opposite way and save money for their families, and their children's education and welfare?

Responsible drinking

Alcohol has been hailed as the oldest, the healthiest and the most popular beverage ever known to mankind. The ancient wise man Plato even declared that, "nothing more excellent nor more valuable than wine has ever been granted to mankind by God". It is a fact that alcoholic beverages can be found in every culture and civilisation throughout human history. In fact, according to recent breakthrough news reported in the *Australian Chinese Daily* (22 March 2021), archaeological finds in excavations at the ancient burial place in Shan Si in 2020 included some brass jars containing scant fluid residues which, on biochemical analysis, turned out to be fruit-based wine, like a modern-day liqueur. Those ancient artifacts and relics have been estimated to be at least two thousand seven hundred years old!

Wine production was first recorded at around 300 BC, but its consumption probably started as early as seven thousand years ago, going off archaeological evidence. This beverage has been promoted every now and again by well-known personalities such as the French medical scientist Louis Pasteur – a household name thanks to it being found on every container of "pasteurised milk" – who echoed with approval the famous remark by Plato quoted above.

Indeed, this sentiment was born out in 1979 when it was found that French people suffered significantly less CVD and MI despite their high cholesterol intake. If any health-conscious reader in their spare time just flips over the pages of a French cookbook, they would be overwhelmed to find page after page of rich ingredients and recipes saturated with butter, cream, mock-cream and full-cream milk. How could the French people consume so much 'unhealthy' food all year round and yet end up winners with lower MI than in most Western countries? It was a sort of anomaly, going against conventional wisdom and so was aptly dubbed the *French Paradox* – destined to be fervently investigated in the subsequent famous Copenhagen Heart Study.

When this study was published in 1995, there was great excitement at the results. They showed that, for the first time in human history, scientific evidence suggested that a moderate amount of wine daily (one or two standard drinks, or 88 to 125ml Australian standard) was beneficial. In fact, it may be that drinking this amount of alcohol is more protective for your heart than being a teetotaller, as statistics show that people who don't drink alcohol at all have double the number of heart attacks that moderate drinkers do.

As heart attack has long been listed as the number one killer in most countries like North America and Australia, it comes as no surprise to see many people proclaiming themselves connoisseurs of wine. After all, a glass or two of good wine at dinner time is most enjoyable. Not only does it complement the food, but it also makes most people more comfortable and communicative socially. Alcohol molecules (ethanol) go to the brain fairly rapidly and depress or dampen the reticular system so that people lose inhibition and start to open up more, becoming increasingly talkative and feeling livelier. So, these are the general benefits of drinking alcohol sensibly and responsibly.

On the other hand, irresponsibly drinking more than this amount will hamper your brain's functionality, and overall, your faculties will be negatively affected. In other words, you lose your sense, your rationality, and your judgement. In this state people may become argumentative or aggressive, leading to involvement with the police, being fined or worse. As is often seen on the TV news, it is not unusual for someone under the influence to crash their car through a fence, into a creek or even into someone's loungeroom. I myself once witnessed the spectacular if absurd and somewhat troubling display of a car halfway up a tree on a road leading out of Melbourne. Tragically, this kind of behaviour even results in the occasional catastrophic head-on, with no survivors emerging from the badly twisted wreckage.

However, when it comes to enjoying the benefits of alcohol, you can become baffled trying to decide what you want to indulge in. Beer? Liqueurs? Spirits? Or wine? Even beer comes in many varieties and brands. The stronger varieties contain about seven per cent alcohol and can bowl you over after a few cans. Healthwise, spirits are generally too strong to consume in large quantities, for most of them contain from thirty to fifty per cent alcohol, like Russian vodka and the Chinese Moutai, which is also very expensive. Even tantalising liqueurs are just spirits with added favours.

So the best choice is wine. Usually, red wines are healthier than their pale cousins, because red wines are fermented along with the grape skins and seeds, while white wine is not. Scientific studies have uncovered a very important fact in wine making which explains why the way reds are made is advantageous. It has been found that the red grape skin and seeds contain rich supplies of plant polyphenols, one of which is resveratrol, which we looked at above. That fact has almost completely unravelled the mystery of the French Paradox.

The logic goes like this – the French traditionally drink wine at every dinner. The resveratrol in the wine mobilises those vitality genes – sirtuins – which protect the CVS (the heart and blood vessels), minimising the harm from excess cholesterols and helping lower mortality from MI. This may well only be part of the explanation as many scientists believe that there are other molecules in the wine that also play a part, along with the resveratrol, but it remains to be established if there are other aspects like different cultural attitudes or ways of managing stress which also play a role.

Nonetheless, this is enough encouragement for many of us to indulge, and one can get dizzy in choosing which wine to drink because of the variety of choices. Just the number of white wines is listed as one hundred and five, while the red (black grapes) amount to at least sixty-one (according to Tom Stevenson's *The World Wine Encyclopaedia*). To help you navigate this bewildering maze, our research tells us that you should go for the red first if health is your main concern. Among the popular are Cabernet Sauvignon, Cabernet Franc, Pinot Noir, Shiraz, Merlot and Grenache. It is best to drink Pinot Noir particularly if the grape has been grown "under stress" because when a plant grows under conditions such as drought, it tends to produce more resveratrol to increase its capacity to survive. However, we are not sure how to really find out which brand of Pinot has got the highest concentration of resveratrol – one to two per cent is the popular guess currently.

One outstanding wine variety is called Canonau, brewed by the shepherds of Sardinia, who drink it themselves every day. You will recall that Sardinia is one of the Blue Zones – those areas which have an unusually high number of centenarians. The vine, suspected to be a Grenache, is native to the island and has not been crossbred with any other vine due to the isolation the location has enjoyed for thousands of years. Most shepherds are happy to grow this variety in their own backyards and brew the wine for their families. Only one of the centenarians has managed to expand his inherited family vineyard to a few hundred acres. He has improved the wine's quality and even won prizes when exporting it to Italy. Investigator Ben Hill reckons it is pretty potent. And it looks like it is a stressed vine because of the higher altitude, and the dry and windy environment it grows in, which may encourage the grapes to produce more concentrated polyphenols that help the shepherds to push back ageing more effectively. Canonau and the characteristic grape it is made from has yet to be studied by any demographers or visiting scientists, but the day it is may not be too far into the future.

Avoiding drug use

Many years ago after my graduation, in the seventies, the only drug abusers in evidence were a few rare Pethidine addicts. By the time I started in general practice in Melbourne in 1973 or thereabouts, their numbers had swollen to the point that you would expect to encounter almost one to two a week. Most addicts are manipulative or skilful in concocting fantastic stories about how much pain they have suffered from past fractures and procedures, and bolster their tales by showing off their old scars. I've even witnessed a few of them roll about on the floor, dramatically clutching their bellies and swearing that that their renal colic was killing them, and nothing short of an injection of Pethidine would help. Others might show you a bottle of diluted blood after having allegedly been to the clinic's toilet, to prove that their kidney stones are causing bloody urine.

After the Pethidine fever died down, a new batch of drug addicts appeared, often smashing windows at the rear of clinics and chemist shops to steal their personal drugs of addiction like amphetamines, opioids and sleeping pills. Fortunately, most of the time, the break-in is spoiled by the alarm and the security guard.

When you sit down and look at the current situation these days, no normal person could escape from the conviction that drugs, invariably those addictive ones, are looming increasingly large as the biggest problem in terms of poisoning society, tearing families apart and tainting the community. These poisonous substances contaminate tens of thousands of young people (as they are usually the targets of drug peddlers) and push them down a black hole of no return. Take a look at Colombia, the drug-cartel capital of the world, for example, it has been reported that murders, killings, kidnappings and battles between government forces and the private armies of the wealthy and powerful cartels has been almost a daily event for years, with hundreds and hundreds of civilians being killed in the crossfire.

Frightening? But the drug peddlers and cartels don't care, as all that concerns them is guarding their territory and the huge profits gained by peddling and selling their toxic wares.

In July 2017, Channel 2 in Sydney reported that the number of drug addicts in the US could be as high as twenty million (Covid-19 positive cases were only six million in September 2020 and generally fatal to a much lesser degree), about two hundred and sixty thousand of whom were on opioids or addictive drugs, legal or illegal.

Due to its long coastline and inadequate surveillance, Australia has long been a soft target for drug cartels and drug dealers. Though these used to be from the Golden Triangle in Southeast Asia, they now come in from all over the world. Just within the last two years, the AFP and the Australia Border Control have busted two of the biggest drug smuggling operations into Sydney ever seen. The first and the largest haul of almost one and a half tonnes of cocaine was seized in February 2017. Unexpectedly, a second assignment followed within a year, of close to 1.3 tonnes of cocaine, and led to the dramatic arrest of a well-known Australian livestock and construction figure Rohan Arnold in a Belgrade luxury hotel by Serbian police, on a tip-off from AFP. The two drug hauls had a combined street value of over a billion Australian dollars: enough to poison a few million young people.

These large-scale seizures, which are front page news, are about drugs confiscated before they could enter the country. There are many more cases in which the smugglers have devised numerous, tricky and ingenious ways via parcels, furniture, toys and even heavy machinery, to fool the border patrol forces and custom officers. It's a great pity that those smugglers misuse their intelligence and time on get-rich-quick schemes, and never pause for a second to consider their victims' welfare. On the other hand, few of us are aware of the existence of the hundreds of small operators setting up their own lab workshops to fiddle around with chemicals and generate unknown amounts of addictive drugs to satisfy the enormous appetite of local drug addicts and fun-seekers. This supply line has also been eagerly pursued by the AFP and the anti-drug agency who have successfully exposed many of them and put the culprits under arrest.

No doubt drug smuggling and border control surveillance is a never-ending war for most countries these days, and as sensible and responsible citizens we must steer away from these addictive poisons. Many youths are naïve and easily persuaded, or plainly conned by their friends or drug peddlers, and so they become the victims of over-dose or death, occurrences which are particularly rife at pop music festivals and entertainment venues, and often gets the drug-takers into the headlines, or straight into the ICU of a nearby hospital for resuscitation. A few of my young patients tell me that they have woken up on the pavement or a park bench after attending a party at their friend's house, and they have absolutely no recollection of what has happened to them, meaning they have had total memory collapse (amnesia) and are surprised that they are still alive! These few lucky young men have recovered from near death and have been able to learn their lesson. They will never again dismiss these powerful drugs as "just a party pill" or just "good fun" to try "for the experience".

In fact, these psychotropic drugs are not only addictive, they can damage the neurons in your brain, damage or break DNA linkages, or even weaken and damage the functions of sirtuins – your longevity gene activators.

Avoid irresponsible gambling

Gambling appears to be a universal habit, deeply rooted in the nature of human beings. One high profile popular form, as everyone knows, is horse racing – which even the English Royal Family involve themselves in, with the Queen's horses participating in many race meetings, including the Derby at Epsom, the Grand National and the Cheltenham Gold Cup.

Australians are no less enthusiastic gamblers than the British. The most famous event, held yearly at Flemington, is the Melbourne Cup – dubbed "the race that stops the nation" as the CBD and most shops close on that particular day, the first Tuesday in November, every year. The race usually starts at about 2:40 p.m. with quite a few horses brought in from overseas. But due to the Covid-19 situation, the post-lockdown after the second wave in Melbourne, and the international border closure in 2020, the cup that year, unlike any other in its history, was a very quiet one – compared with 2019's where eighty-one thousand fans attended. According to a horse psychologist, the horses, particularly the thoroughbreds who are said to be a more sensitive animal, would have been more relaxed without the raucous crowd! It is a tough race over a distance of three thousand two hundred metres, but is rewarded by a whopping eight million dollars in prize money. And the Caufield Cup meeting is run before the Melbourne Cup and the Oak's Day race (a lady's day) afterward. Altogether, it is a four-day Cup Carnival, normally a really entertaining and riveting event.

Sydney, which has been trying to catch up when it comes to horse racing, has got its own event, the Sydney Cup, which has been running annually since 1862 (just one year less than the Melbourne Cup) but it has never been able to pose a formidable challenge to the Melbourne Cup in terms of interest and prestige. Instead, Sydneysiders are much more fervent about water sports, particularly the yearly Sydney to Hobart yacht race – another major event bound to attract much heavy betting and rich prize money.

Next in line would be greyhound racing – a less glamorous but no less popular spectator sport than horse racing. It was once banned in NSW recently, after alleged cruelty and inhuman treatment of some of the animals was discovered by inspectors. The situation has since been rectified and these exciting races have got back on track again.

Even the tiny island of Hong Kong has been hustling to catch up and has done well by operating two well-planned racecourses – the famous Happy Valley Racecourse on Hong Kong Island and the Sha Tin Racecourse in the New Territory opposite the island. It is no surprise that the Chinese are big horseracing fans and big gamblers. They have recruited (or enticed) quite a few famed Australian jockeys to train the local Chinese jockeys (the younger brother of one of my high school friends being one of them).

The Chinese are heavily addicted to gambling. They are well known to frequent Macao's casinos and made the front page as "high-rollers" in the infamous inquiry into Melbourne's Crown Casino conducted in 2020 by the NSW Independent Liquor and Gaming Authority (ILGA), which found that the Crown group had committed a string of governance and risk management failures – admitted by Ms Coonan, the Crown Resort chairperson who took serious note of these mistakes and promised to implement a stronger anti-money laundering strategy and improve the company's culture. James Packer (son of Kerry Packer, the richest man in Australia and famous for a gambling loss of twenty-six million dollars at a UK casino many years ago) is the biggest shareholder, owning thirty-six per cent of the Crown. He is also a background director, and was closely questioned via Zoom during the inquiry while recuperating on his twenty million dollar super yacht off Sydney harbour.

The ILGA inquiry is a follow-up investigation by the crime watchdog AUSTRAC which occurred when investigative journalists from the *Sydney Morning Herald* and *Sixty Minutes* uncovered the fact that the large high-roller "junket" tour organiser Suncity (which is run by the alleged former Macau triad member Alvin Chau) was reported to have operated a private gaming room at the Crown Casino in Melbourne and over five and a half million dollars in cash had been found stored in a cupboard in a private room in 2018. Soon after, chief CEO Ken Barton and three directors of the Crown resigned in

February 2021, reportedly farewelled with settlements of multiple millions.

This dirty linen is only the tip of an iceberg of corruption. There are many dark sides to gambling and drug running which are mixed up with many other vices and crimes in the underworld. It goes without saying that money laundering and drug running are as bread and butter to most of the world's famous casinos. It is a never-ending story, and they will probably never be cleaned up – like cancers and chronic diseases, these dark associations are deep-seated and incurable.

It is probably harmless to go to casinos with your family or friends just for the sake of entertainment; but it is an entirely different matter if you go to those establishments alone regularly when you feel lonely, depressed and bored, because then you have no one to advise you to stop emptying your pocket, to help you resist the urge to keep playing at the table or at the poker machine (which is aptly dubbed a "one arm bandit"). Don't forget that only high rollers can afford to play big because they are rich and some of them are spending big to launder money they have earned from unlawful sources. We ordinary working people should always be mindful of the Cantonese saying that the worst four sinful habits in life are "prostitution, gambling, alcohol addiction and opium or drug taking".

In Hong Kong, we used to get a laugh from a story about a habitual gambler who went to Macau (the Monte Carlo of the Orient) to gamble in the casino (somehow, Hong Kong has none). Naturally, he lost heavily but his urge to keep gambling had overcome his sense, and he wouldn't quit for anything. As credit cards were unheard of in those days the only way for him to continue was to go to the pawn shop to pawn his valuables: watch, gold chain (no mobile in those days) and his suit. Later he was seen on the returning boat dressed only in his underpants – his last valuable! Everything else has been lost. This hilarious story was well known by most Hong Kong people at the time.

Today, unfortunately, the story would be very different because of that plastic card and the ease with which money can be transferred electronically. You could quickly lose your wages for that day, and your life savings would not take long to vanish either. The next thing that usually happens is borrowing from friends, relatives and business partners. Then you could lose your car and your house, and naturally your spouse. Many addicted gamblers go even further and swindle large sums from their employer until they are discovered and end up in jail or as suicides.

We have to remind ourselves that gambling addiction is a disease: a form of mental illness, similar to addiction to drugs and any vice. If you think you are in danger, then it is best to consult a psychiatrist, a relevant government agency, or a private gambling advisory service for proper treatment early, before it is too late.

Remain connected

Human beings have been gregarious animals ever since they first appeared on this earth. We like to gather together socially, live in groups and communicate with others so that we can share work, information and other benefits, and that is the key for us to survive and improve.

The closest relationships are, of course, those of the basic family unit composed of parents and children. This may be further extended to all relatives and the wider clan. And not to not forget your workmates and colleagues if you work in a city office, or your co-workers, neighbours and villagers if you work in the country in a small town or village. It won't take long before you become familiar with each other and form a circle of working friends. Australians are comparatively more friendly and easy to get along with than other people.

It is of huge benefit to connect with other human beings as much as possible. It is even more gratifying to be part of a circle of friends who are able to contact each other anytime to talk about life: how the children are going with school, what family events are coming up, matters of nutrition, home cooking, the state of the world (like the situation with the pandemic at the time of writing) or what's happening in your own neck of the woods. Such frequent discussions and exchanges of opinion are enjoyed by everybody; we all need to share our experiences and feelings, rather than being isolated with our thoughts bottled up to some degree. There will, of course, be extreme introverts reading this who think, *not me*, but most people need some kind of network to live a fulfilled life, even if it is only a partner or a few family members and friends.

Obviously, a great many people see the benefits of this and have wasted no time in getting onto their electronic devices to communicate with each other during the severe lockdowns which occurred since March 2020. During that period, there was an increase of over one hundred per cent in mobile phone usage! You cannot blame electronic gadget salesmen for laughing all the way to the bank, and the brand name electronic shops have witnessed their stock go sky high on the share market too!

So keep connected to the world, keep communicating with your family, your group, your business associates. You won't go wrong – in fact, it will be the opposite. By utilising and training your brain to prevent the insidious onslaught of Alzheimer's and other mental diseases, you are literally helping yourself to push back ageing.

Learn how to relax and sleep well

As we all know, the society we are living in, particularly in the CBD of a big city, is highly competitive and unforgiving. Everyone is rushing about in the city, and noisy cars, buses and trams seem to come from nowhere on a collision course. There are a lot of headaches: tension from rushing to the bus stop or train platform, preparing to face the jostling of the peak-hour, groups of students who never cease chatting and laughing, not to mention emitting the occasional shriek for no good reason. No wonder most nine-to-five workers return home tired, if not totally exhausted, and can lose the energy to socialise with their family. Instead, many head to the lounge chair and the six o'clock TV news.

Even those who drive daily may not fare any better. Peak-hour traffic can be horrific even without the occasional accident which brings everything to a halt, sometimes making major roads unnegotiable for hours. There may be clogging at a bottle-neck, or an unseasonal flooding of the road, or a crash in a tunnel which can keep the traffic at a standstill for what seems like an eternity. There's nothing you can do: even using your mobile phone may get you fined. Finding a parking space sometimes is not the easiest task either, and once you do you can still get a ticket if you have merely misread the often ambiguous parking signs. And those who travel by car need still more energy to concentrate and perform well once they have arrived at work safe and sound. That is to say nothing of the stress faced by those workers whose jobs involve spending all day in traffic, like the drivers of buses, taxis and all kinds of delivery vehicles. And then there are those who combine this with a job high in other stressors, like paramedics and officers of the law!

All that headache, tension and worry is harmful and it is best to minimise and manage it before it can become chronic and habitual. These are the harbingers of mental unease and illness if you do not ameliorate them or channel them elsewhere to restore your mental wellness. These psychological factors can cut your life short by a few years.

So the question is – how best to relax your body and mind? One ancient solution to this age-old goal is the practise of meditation, which has been promoted by ancient wise men, religious leaders and their followers, monks and priests. It has been practised in different forms in every major religion, both in the East and the West. It even influenced the Beatles in the sixties when they learnt Transcendental Meditation under the Indian yogi Maharishi Mahesh Yogi.

Meditation may simply be described as the practice of techniques such as mindfulness, or focusing on a word or phrase (a mantra) or some other form of mental process which conditions consciousness to be more disciplined, thereby allowing the practitioner to attain a state of greater lucidity, coherence and equilibrium. The popularity and practice of meditation has recently become widespread, as can be seen by the numerous studios, self-help programmes and self-proclaimed therapy centres offering it to clients. The reason for this is that meditation is very simple to learn, and is probably the cheapest form of therapy in the world. It has been studied by Professor Herbert Benson of Harvard University who coined the term "relaxation response", which means that an individual's body can overcome tension and anxiety with their harmful effects such as increased pulse rates, high BP and metabolic rates through properly trained and disciplined relaxation.

It is the most affordable therapy because there are no drugs or equipment required. All you have to do is to sit in a quiet spot for about ten minutes, close your eyes and concentrate on one thought, idea or word, and loosen up your body (and muscles) from your feet up to your upper body, neck and face. The important point is to practise regularly so that your body becomes used to this new biological response and will be more efficient in its performance. After practising meditation regularly for a while, people feel calmer and their muscles are more relaxed. Their mood is enhanced, they enjoy improved digestion and suffer less from everyday stress.

The major Melbourne newspaper *The Age* reported on 9 January 2005 that a team of scientists at the University of Wisconsin, led by Richard J. Davidson, had conducted a series of brain scans on meditating Tibetan monks. He discovered that gamma waves, which are unusually fast and powerful, are particularly active, well organised and coordinated in the rains of senior monks who are expert meditators, compared to those in novices' brains. Apparently, gamma waves indicate the mental process of those who have achieved higher mental activity and awareness. In another study, Davidson and his team discovered that the left frontal cortex, a region associated with happiness, positive thought and emotion, appears to be most intensely active when an individual is meditating.

Now let's look at another important matter in our lives – sleep – which is just one part of our daily journey, an essential break after the demands of the waking day. Most people don't seem to be aware of the fact that we spend one third of our life in bed, or on average eight hours per day. As we are all different in our body chemistry, so too are our sleep patterns and the amount of time we spend asleep. Some sleep "like a baby" and it is difficult to wake them up, others toss and turn all night with insomnia, or perhaps due to medical problems. For example, the British WWII Prime Minister Winston Churchill slept only five hours, the "Iron Lady" Margaret Thatcher reportedly even less. On the opposite side is the genius physicist Albert Einstein who needed over ten hours of sleep! Most people fall between these extremes, sleeping six to eight hours of a night. As a rule, babies and younger people need more sleep to compensate for their higher metabolic rate of growth, and need fewer hours than more elderly people, except those who still work hard physically.

The reason why we sleep, like most mammals, is because we have a built-in biological clock which matches the circadian rhythm controlled by a hormone called Melatonin which is excreted from the pineal gland in the brain. Our sleep is usually composed of two stages – REM (Rapid Eye Movement) and NREM (non-REM). REM is the dreaming stage that is marked by increased brain activity, while NREM is the deepest stage and does the most to refresh you physically, right down to every single cell in your body. You need both stages alternating with each other in a cyclical manner to derive the maximum benefit, and for your body to be completely recovered and your energy restored.

Chronic lack of sleep can lead many unpleasant effects like a lack of energy, listlessness, a loss of interest in socialising, a loss of confidence, depression and habitual drug taking. Sometimes this is only in the form of sleeping pills but that is bad enough. To break the insomnia-sleeping-pill cycle, the first remedy should be meditation, and you need to observe sleep hygiene by ceasing smoking and drinking alcohol, coffee, tea and cola-type drinks that contain caffeine, and taking harmful stimulant-type drugs. You should also avoid discussing serious problems and worries before sleep, avoid exciting TV programmes as well, and get rid of any noisy gadgets in your bedroom such as wall-clocks.

Try to follow a healthy routine of going to bed at the same time every night after ten minutes of meditation, and to avoid having too many late nights through going out. It is also helpful to get up at about the same time every morning. After a while, you won't need an alarm clock to remind you to get up – your biological clock and natural circadian rhythm will take over.

If you are inclined to be an active person and not used to sitting quietly to practise meditation, then the modified Chinese martial art called Tai Chi may appear more attractive to you as it is sometimes described as a form of "moving meditation".

Try Tai Chi, also called "shadow boxing", is an ancient form of martial art established about eight hundred years ago. It is a kind of slow-moving exercise that can also be utilised as a defensive fighting art when it is sped up. It was first developed by a general in the Ming Dynasty and named (after him) "Chang's style". Since then, the style has been modified and named after each master. So you have the Young, Ng and Wu styles, too. However, they are basically quite similar and vary mainly in speed and posture.

The basic movements start at twenty-four and extend up to over a hundred. You only need the basic twenty-four movements to get the hang of it and it is most important to practise regularly. The principle is to adopt a stable posture with both legs bent, your spine straight, and move slowly with purpose, paired with "abdominal breathing" to help you concentrate your mind while relaxing your entire body. The posture strengthens the legs and the core in particular, while the movements help keep the body supple by stretching and twisting in different directions as if dealing with a horde of attackers from all sides in extreme slow motion. You can get onto the net to order a demonstration video of this popular relaxing practice, or to find out where classes are available locally, as well as the hours and the cost. Tai chi not only helps to break the insomnia-sleeping-pill cycle, it has many other health benefits.

Tai Chi is an ideal warm-up exercise for anyone from young children to ninety-year-olds because of the gentle, continuous, free-flowing nature of its movements, which involve most of the joints and muscles of your body. It is extremely suitable as part of a rehabilitation programme – ideally coordinated with physiotherapy and hydrotherapy – for people recovering from injuries, medical operations, or after bone fractures or multiple injuries after a motor car accident, for instance. However, I have yet to see this included in the Medicare Schedule of Resources that help the disabled to recover as early as possible.

Tai Chi is beneficial for your heart and cardiovascular system. The smooth gentle motions which incorporate the use of all of your limbs without jerky, violent action will be most welcome to your heart. Furthermore, the regular deep abdominal breathing will guarantee better oxygen saturation of the blood flow in the lungs.

Naturally such Tai Chi exercises, if carried out regularly, could be the most ideal therapy for asthmatics due to the regular, controlled, deep abdominal breathing they stimulate. For a long time, knowledgeable doctors have understood this secret and have devoted time to educating their asthmatic patients on the virtues of regular deep breathing practise which involves using the diaphragm more fully, as in abdominal breathing, rather than the shallow breathing which is caused by the use of the rather weak rib cage muscles. Because of this same principle, asthmatics will fare better if they swim regularly.

Tai Chi will give you a stronger yet more flexible spine because the key point in Tai Chi movements is that the trunk (spine) drives all limb movements while it remains a central anchorage point. Of course, the brain initiates this movement, but the practitioner uses the spine as a central pivoting pillar. Many other health benefits include enhanced function such as better balance and coordination, increased endurance, sharper reflexes, improved digestion and GIT function, and better flexibility in practically every joint.

For well over a thousand years, since the Tang dynasty and long before modern Western medicine emerged, Tai Chi has been included among the holistic therapeutic health practices of the East, together with herbal medicine and acupuncture. So, go for Tai Chi if you are sick, and do even more Tai Chi if you are well!

Increase your intake of vegetables and fruit
In 1981, the US Congress commissioned two famed British epidemiologists, Richard Doll and Richard Peto, to study and evaluate why Americans suffered such a high rate of CVD, cancer and stroke, with just the CVD death rate alone being seventeen times higher than in China, or roughly three thousand MI deaths per day. After careful surveys, the two scientists drafted a report to Congress, which indicated that the major culprit was Americans' unhealthy lifestyle, involving tobacco smoking and a diet dominated by excess animal meat and fatty food which pushed up their blood cholesterol and therefore their MI rate. They strongly recommended that the American people consume more vegetables and fruits instead of their regular fatty fare, while taking up regular exercise.

However, at the time of the survey, and for a long time since to this very day, not more than four to five per cent of Americans take regular exercise seriously, nor do they seek to lead a healthy lifestyle, the benefits of which have already been described at length above. We will discuss the immensely important topic of diet in Chapter Seven.

The International Heart Study on twenty-nine thousand patients from fifty-two countries drew the astonishing conclusion that ninety to ninety-four per cent of all CVD is due to unhealthy lifestyle. The survey also found that an unhealthy diet was an associated factor in ninety per cent of the cases of gastric and colon cancer. This simply underlines the fact that we must remind ourselves to do the right thing in life and follow a healthy lifestyle as detailed earlier, in order to stimulate the longevity genes to push back the ageing process which is, unfortunately, often accompanied by quite a few unpleasant diseases, if not deadly cancers.

Consider "wonder drugs"

On the other hand, we can now enlist some "wonder pills", which through sheer hard work and solid research have been discovered over the last two decades by the smart brains in reputable labs all over the world. Often the experiments which test the new theories are based on inspired observations at subcellular levels far beyond our understanding, or even our imagination, because subcellular phenomena occur on the nanoscale.

One of the difficulties that scientists researching longevity face is that getting results from experiments on lab animals takes a long time, and they often fail or have to be repeated many times to be considered conclusive. When any significant result is obtained and published in a reputable journal, it needs confirmation from other good labs before the findings are approved and recognised by the global research community. I discovered this myself when I conducted research work in the past: it all involved hard work, boring procedures and scanning many journals for relevant information.

After the important discovery of the longevity gene activator, Professor Sinclair has subsequently uncovered a few more pathways to longevity, including enzymes that could prolong the lives of lab animals by up to fifty per cent, which is equivalent to adding thirty to forty years of life in human terms. What is more amazing, and this has been confirmed in other independent labs, is that the genetic and epigenetic mechanisms operating the survival circuit in everything from Homo sapiens to the lowly simple yeast cell or the primordial organism has hardly changed over the four million years since the first primitive organisms first appeared on earth! This is truly incredible.

The following are the major wonder drugs discovered. When taken as instructed, they appear to activate our Longevity genes. For the first time in human history, instead of needing to rely on CR or exercise, they can be used to do all those repair jobs on DNA, turning genes on and off to protect us against ageing and all its unwelcome companions: CVD, stroke, NIDDM, cancers, Alzheimers and osteoarthritis.

Resveratrol
This famous chemical is one of the plant chemicals collectively called polyphenols. It was first reported by Sinclair's lab in 2006, shocking the scientific world because of its proven ability to activate the longevity genes (SIRTs from one to seven as found in mammals) and helping to unravel the "French Paradox". This is because this enzyme, contained in red wine, appeared to be the key chemical which reduces the rich cholesterol in French cuisine so that regular drinkers suffer far less MI compared to non-drinkers, or to the citizens of other nations.

In July 2008, Sinclair et al. reported that resveratrol-treated mice were found to have much lower rates of CVD, as well as reduced cholesterol and blood sugar, stronger and thicker bones and a longer lifespan, even on a high-calorie diet. Yet they did not gain weight and showed more energy and endurance on the treadmill. One of them even broke the record by running three kilometres and damaged the lab treadmill, which had never happened before. This was because the mice on resveratrol had increased mitochondria in their muscles which made them more athletic, yet without them having to do the athletic training usually required. Meanwhile the control group of mice not treated with resveratrol all died off within their usual lifespan.

The only problem with resveratrol is that you don't get enough from red wine unless the vine is grown under stressful conditions like dry weather or strong sun. The best variety of wine, as far as its natural levels of resveratrol goes, is Pinot noir. Even Pinot noir only produces one to five milligrams per litre, or even less if not grown in a "stressful" environment.

By a bit of luck, a man called Peter Voigt, a newcomer to grape growing on the Mornington Peninsula in the state of Victoria in Australia, tried his hand at growing the Pinot noir vine without much success, and most of the grape were harvested but unsold, partly due to the wine glut around the world at the time. He did not know what to do with it and left tanks of pinot wine, skin and seed for weeks. When he saw the thick dark mix it had turned into, he decided to stir it into a juice and was able to extract the polyphenol. At about that time he also heard about Sinclair's discovery of resveratrol and contacted him to offer his concentrated grape extract. Sinclair immediately tried it out on mice and was happy to find that Peter Voigt's extract contained more than seven times the resveratrol that normal red wine does. It was as good as the pharmaceutical version of resveratrol. So it turned out Peter Voigt's frustrating business was transformed into a promising commercial venture and his hard work led to a happy ending after all.

As other scientists around the globe have by now realised that a simple molecule like resveratrol can activate our longevity genes, and that there are over a thousand types of polyphenols in the plant kingdom, so many centres have switched their research activities to investigating those wonder substances. This study of plant chemicals, or phytochemicals, is relatively new, yet we humans have been living with plants, vegetables and fruits as long as humans have been on earth, without paying enough attention to the protective effects of phytochemicals.

If you take a stroll in the market, your eye will inevitably be attracted to the eye-pleasing displays of colourful fruits: beautiful strawberries, logan berries, deep red tomatoes and persimmons, bright yellow-green fresh bananas, reddish shiny delicious apples, attractive freshly cut bright green broccoli and bitter melons. Walking back home, we might also take time to appreciate those brilliant, showy flowers in your neighbours' gardens. And where I live, in Sydney, during spring, large, graceful Jacarandas with their vibrant purple flowers are in full bloom everywhere, carpeting the ground below with colour. Surely Australia is a "lucky country", in particular for those of us living in Sydney, which is frequently ranked in the top three of the world's most liveable cities (with Melbourne usually in spot number one). The climate is so mild and comfortable that it is as close to the ideal as could be imagined, for most people, and the wonderful fine white sand and deep blue sea of iconic Bondi Beach, reflecting the heavenly blue sky, is only minutes away from the city's fringe – an instant paradise for the water baby. And in winter, yet another paradise is only a short car trip from greater Sydney in the Perisher Valley, where snow lovers can frolic to their heart's content and skiing enthusiasts can enjoy their favourite pastime.

Further research on resveratrol has revealed that it is not very potent or soluble so as to be readily absorbed in our gut. However, scientists have theorised that similar chemicals might be able to do a better job and went in search of these desirable substances. And indeed, Sinclair's team, after pursuing the problem relentlessly, managed to find another nineteen SIRT 1-activating compounds. Seventeen of the nineteen are polyphenols – collectively called STAC (SIRT 1 activating compounds). The two that particularly impressed Sinclair are called SRT 1720 and SRT 2104. Of course, the code names don't mean much to the layman and the non-scientist but I have included them in case the reader wishes to engage in further research on them.

Nicotinamide adenosine nucleotide (NAD)

NAD, or vitamin B3, is another STAC which has been discovered. It is found in a lot of food (please refer to Chapter Seven) and is made by our cells converting the precursor, nicotinamide mononucleotide, which is the same chemical but in slightly modified form to be better utilised by the body, into NAD. This STAC has been found to be involved in not less than five hundred different enzyme reactions in our bodies. It is an energy booster, capable of boosting all seven sirtuins by serving as fuel that enables them to utilise more energy in the important task of removing the acetyl group from histones (the protein that forms the core of DNA packaging) so that genes can be turned on and off more quickly and efficiently. Basically, they help protect your health more swiftly and push back ageing faster, thereby keeping you younger.

The vitamin B3 in our body is boosted by exercise and healthy eating, but the effectiveness of this alone may slowly decrease with age and need to be supplemented. Dosages come in 500mg tablets, which normally need to be taken twice a day in order to adequately keep the longevity genes active enough to push back ageing. Hopefully, in the future some scientist or pharmaceutical company will find a NAD super-booster that will confer more energy on the seven sirtuins to help push back ageing even better.

Rapamycin

If the name sounds like an antibiotic to you, you are not wrong. It is an extract of the secretion from a bacteria named actinobacterium. It was discovered on a scientific expedition to the remote volcanic location of Rapa Island which is situated 2300 miles West of Chile. A chemist on the team discovered two unusual properties: one is anti-fungal, which makes it good for tinea and ordinary athlete's foot-type fungus infections of no great importance; but the other quite unexpected property is that rapamycin functions as a suppressor of our immune system and needs to be prescribed with caution. Nonetheless, it is certainly another useful weapon for transplant surgeons who in the 1960s had been frustrated by the high rate of transplant-failures due to the new organ being rejected by its recipient.

At that time, kidney transplants (human renal allografts) were one of the hottest topics in North America, and Dr Tolnai (a renal pathologist) and I had partnered together to study the morphological changes in human renal allografts of twenty-seven chronic renal-failure patients. They were being treated with a kidney-transplant procedure at the two main teaching hospitals of Ottawa (Ottawa General and Civic General hospitals) in the Canadian capital, between 1966 and 1970.

Immunosuppressors were widely used and consisted of Imuran, cortisone and actinomycin D (most probably related to rapamycin because it is an extract from actinobacterium). The changes in the renal allografts examined showed a wide range of histological damage from homograft rejection causing severe inflammatory cellular infiltration, tubular necrosis leading to infarction (death) of the graft, and PAS material deposition in the glomeruli (the filtration units of kidney). In the case of homograft rejection, adjustment of the dose in some of the repeat biopsies appeared to work well after immunosuppression therapy and the graft survived. I had the honour to present the research paper at the Ontario pathologists' meeting, pointing out that renal biopsies were a very useful aid to help the clinician in adjusting the dose of immunosuppressant in order to reverse the rejection and save the transplanted kidneys, whether they were from a cadaver (a dead body) or live graft.

In recent years, this same chemical, rapamycin, re-emerged with another surprise for the scientific world, when it was discovered to be the most powerful compound when it comes to life extension. Fancy that – from being a nondescript secretion from an actinobacterium thought to have simple anti-fungal use to being promoted for use as a very promising immunosuppressant, and now a very potent pill to push back ageing! The effectiveness of rapamycin was indicated in an experiment in Sinclair's lab in which ageing mice given small doses of rapamycin had about nine to fourteen per cent longer lives. This amounts to about a decade of additional healthy life in human terms.

Metformin

I would be very disappointed if only a few of my readers are familiar with metformin because of the fact that diabetes mellitus (DM) is now the fastest-growing disease, and metformin has been the first-line anti-diabetic medication for years. It is cheap, effective and has very few unpleasant side effects. It has also recently been incorporated into the treatment for polycystic ovary syndrome (PCOS) and I have witnessed several of my patients recover and successfully conceive a child after treatment. This is amazing, as PCOS seems to take root from an unhealthy lifestyle and hormonal imbalance (overweight, obesity, failure to ovulate, infertility, hirsutism and acne) – not unlike the notorious metabolic syndrome. All of this makes it difficult to treat.

As mentioned above, the rate of DM is rapidly rising thanks to the tendency of people to indulge their sweet tooth with an unlimited supply of soft drinks and energy drinks which all contain a high percentage of sugar – up to fifteen per cent – rich, tempting sweets and desserts, and the plethora of sugary goodies on the shelves of supermarkets. Because none of these is essential and DM is frequently merely the result of overindulgence, it is frequently described as one of the "diseases of affluence".

Diabetes mellitus is classified as either type I (insulin dependent, or IDDM) or type II (non- insulin dependent: NIDDM) with the former happening in younger age groups, often after a viral infection which has damaged the pancreas, or is now more commonly regarded as an auto-immune disease, like pernicious anaemia, thyroiditis, glomerulonephritis (inflammation of the renal filtration units) and multiple sclerosis (MS, damaged wrapping sheath of nerves).

Interestingly, Dr Colin Campbell in his twenty years' research has emphatically pointed out that the further you live away from the equator, the more auto-immune disease you will encounter. He explains that the cause could well be that fragments of cow milk protein from incomplete digestion pass into the blood stream and are mistaken for foreign proteins by the immune system, thereby incurring its wrath. If these fragments look like pancreatic cells, they will be destroyed by the T-cells (the immune cells). Campbell has found that Finnish children consume up to sixteen times more milk than Japanese children, and theorises that this is why IDDM is thirty-six times more common in Finland than in Japan. This truly incredible statistic is surely worth more study by immunologists.

Campbell has also collected data showing MS is up to one hundred times more prevalent in the far north than at the equator – another incredible fact. So Campbell strongly recommends parents feed their new-born infants on breast milk or soymilk for at least six months, and preferably for some years thereafter, until the baby's immune system becomes more mature and stable. The recommendations make sense, but the public needs to be re-educated if this new concept is going to influence common practice.

The second type of DM is the more prevalent type II, or NIDDM, which used to be regarded as a malady that the older-age group is prone to. It is impossible to miss the mushrooming of coffee lounges, eateries, supermarkets and other venues stocked to the roof with soft drinks, confectionary and other unhealthy sugar-laden food. Even an eight-year-old can tell you why more and more people are getting NIDDM – the evidence is far too obvious, but a lot of people seems to be born with a sweet tooth, and they find it hard not to over-indulge, regardless of whether they may soon suffer the consequences mentioned below.

In Australia, a recent national survey confirms that the instance of known DM sufferers numbers close to four per cent of the population. In addition to this, there are another ten to sixteen per cent of potential DM sufferers according to the GTT (glucose-tolerance test), means that the total is between seventeen to twenty-three per cent of the total population being affected. That's close to one in every four persons in our society. The latest news is that about three hundred new DM cases per day are reported, which amounts to there being almost one new DM sufferer created every five minutes. Such data, no doubt, can equally be applied to most Western countries, and it is sadly becoming a global issue.

All these are not just numbers, percentage, and statistics; they are real people, many of whom are in the dark about the harm DM could do to them in the short term, and, more frighteningly, they are also ignorant of the more devastating damage they may face in the long term, as described below.

Firstly, they will suffer impaired peripheral circulation, causing a commonly known condition called gangrene (infection following the death of the tissue). It usually starts with small arteries in a single toe becoming blocked. Due to the blockage a very painful ulcer forms which alerts the sufferer so they often seek medical aid immediately. However, when it comes to NIDDM, the pain-sensitive nerves in the toe or foot have lost their function, so that the pain is not severe enough for the patient to seek medical help. Gangrene will not heal without improvement of the patient's overall NIDDM, and the sufferer usually has to undergo one of the three to four thousand amputations performed every year in Australia. Thirty percent are of toes, in ten per cent of operations feet are removed, and the rest involve a major part of the limb at the knee joint or even higher up.

Although there has not been sufficient research to explain why small peripheral arteries become blocked in chronic cases of NIDDM, I found some interesting pathology when conducting over three hundred autopsies on deceased patients in the Ottawa General Hospital – many of whom had died of MI. What aroused my curiosity was that some of the coronary arteries, kidney arteries and large leg arteries consistently showed much opaque, gelatinous material filling a significant amount of the arteries' interior space. When the stained histology sections were returned to me, the jelly filling, all stained pink by PAS dye during preparation, indicated that the stuff could be carbohydrates, which is in fact a compound of sugar.

And now, naturally, my educated guess is that NIDDM, being a metabolic disorder of glucose and carbohydrate, may cause abnormal carbohydrates or proteins to slowly build up on the arterial walls, like that PAS-stained pink jelly, until one day enough has accumulated to completely block the blood supply to the toes, feet and legs (causing gangrene); or where it affects the kidneys, and the coronary artery it is a co-culprit setting off a case of MI – a heart attack.

This seems to be the missing piece of the jigsaw puzzle that we doctors have for years been told by cardiologists: diabetic patients having a heart attack suffer chest pain to a lesser degree than those without diabetes. When we recall that diabetics do not feel much pain from a gangrenous toe, then we can consider the cause identical: the arteries are blocked by the gelatin, damaging the pain sense of nerves so that their MI pain is much less severe.

Secondly, in diabetic neuropathy, the peripheral nerves are particularly affected so that they have reduced functionality. Therefore, it doesn't register when the toe or foot is squeezed into a tight shoe, no pain is felt when a blister forms and bursts, nor is any discomfort experienced even when an ulcer forms, becomes infected, and ultimately becomes gangrenous. Some of the luckier patients have found out about their condition when their complaint of feeling numb in their foot or leg is investigated and their lab test shows a high level of sugar, clinching the diagnosis. Once the problem has been discovered and they adjust their habits, they may slowly recover optimal control of their blood sugar, but there is no guarantee of that.

Thirdly, in about thirty per cent of chronic NIDDM patients, the kidneys may gradually become damaged until diabetic renopathy develops which, although not a common condition or an acute onset problem, could still be a serious disease which the NIDDM patient can ill afford to ignore. It has been found that a chronic diabetic state upsets the kidneys and causes the blood pressure to rise significantly. DM combined with high blood pressure will damage the kidneys, and continuously neglecting to control both will lead to kidney failure. Once the kidneys have failed, nothing can help except dialysis or a transplant. Both are troublesome remedies – the former involves changing your blood every two days for life, and the latter is rather expensive, plus you have to wait for a suitable donor to turn up.

Fourthly, a prolonged state of high glucose levels in the blood and tissue can result in some proteins becoming coated with glucose, the result being glycation: proteins in the body becoming caramelised to form AGE (advanced glycation end-products). AGE impairs immune defence and leads to a high incidence of cancer. The degree of damage can be measured by a simple blood test called HbA1c which it is recommended DM patients have every three months. To avoid AGE, you need to steer away from foods like that tasty Chinese-style roast duck created when hot flames lick the fowl's sweetly marinated skin, causing the sugar to combine with the skin proteins to form the glycation products. Similarly, damaging proteins can also be produced when roasting pork and chicken and on the good old Aussie BBQ.

Anecdotal news began circulating in China years ago about the rampant number of cases of oesophageal cancer, which like liver cancer and cancer of the nose, is common in China. It was rumoured to be due to the over-consumption of roast duck, and warnings were issued from the health authorities that lovers of this food should exercise more restraint!

Fifthly – diabetic retinopathy. This is one of the most dreaded complications from prolonged DM or poorly controlled NIDDM, both of which can damage the blood vessels of the retina, causing haemorrhage and exudation (meaning fluid leaking or seeping through blood vessel walls) which results, naturally, in the deterioration of vision. It can be treated, but equally important is immediate control of the blood-sugar level. The victim sometimes fails to recognise the disease or is in denial in regard to it.

Many years ago, not long after I had joined the Glenroy Road Clinic in Melbourne, one of the receptionists, a rather plump girl who was generally a good worker, was noticed behaving somewhat erratically. She did things which were not at all typical for her, like misfiling patient record cards (this was back in the days before computers when those four-by-eight inch cards were the popular way to keep records). She even began to bump into the other staff on occasion, which was something she had never done before. All those minor incidents were initially blamed on lack of sleep and worrying about her sick mum, and understandably aroused a lot of attention and sympathy from the other staff. One day she hit her head on one of those metal filing cabinets that had not been pushed back after filing, as often happened at busy sessions. Although it was only a very light blow, this girl just lost her balance and fell to the floor, which was carpet, fortunately. It was only then that she admitted that she had suffered from NIDDM for a long time and her vision was becoming increasingly blurry. That was it, she had to quit her job and get proper laser treatment on her retina immediately, rather than attempting to hide her illness in order to retain her job.

Metformin is biguanide – a refined extract from the chemical guanidine discovered by French scientist Jean Sterne, who was curious about the therapeutic effect of a popular medicinal plant called "French lilac"– a lovely purple flowering plant. Now, just imagine – an important pill made from a flower, is it possible? Or is it a fantasy?

Well, just listen to the WHO, which estimates that eighty-five per cent of the world's population depends directly on plants as medicine! Eighty-five per cent, not just 8.5 per cent! And, over twenty-five per cent of our current prescription drugs, and nearly *all* of our recreational substances come from the plant kingdom, the common ones being caffeine in coffee, theophylline and many chemicals in tea, cocaine and marijuana, also called cannabis. This herb has been in use since ancient times, but was criminalised for much of the twentieth century. Now it has been officially sanctioned to be grown in Tasmania for medical uses, in a project jointly developed and managed with Canada. How profoundly human attitudes change over time! The latest news is that you can buy cannabis oil for migraine and painful conditions over the counter, without prescription! And there are now hemp-infused drinks of all sorts on supermarket shelves!

In mid-March 2021, professor Michael Vagg, Dean of Pain Medicine at ANZCA (Australia's peak pain-advisory body), strongly advised doctors not to prescribe medicinal cannabis to treat patients with chronic pain, saying that there is no robust evidence to prove cannabinoid products are effective, while proponents including the TGA (Therapeutic Goods Authority), like the FDA in the US, say the products should be given the benefit of doubt. So far, the TGA has already approved its one hundred thousandth medicinal cannabis application, most which have been prescribed for chronic pain. Well, maybe cannabis will prove its worth in chronic pain with longer usage.

Quite a few EU countries have shown intense interest in herbal medicine. Germany in particular has established a government agency called the Commission to Assess Herbal Products. The UK has its famous Kew Gardens with a large area growing medicinal herbs. Some Okinawans (the island with the most concentrated centenarian concentration in the world) have managed to discover many herbs and medicinal plants of great nutritional and medicinal value. They developed this tradition further and established a herbal farm connected to a special health-food restaurant – what a pleasant enterprise to attract tourists!

But herbal medicine has never been an easy field of study. You must be prepared to spend a great deal of time checking the specimens you collect from the fields, riversides and hills and comparing them with the illustrations in reference books of medicinal plants (well-presented works are pretty scarce in the days since my late father carried out major research into them). You shouldn't expect to earn any money to supplement your lost time and income. My father, an ENT Professor, was just one of those stubborn scholars with only one single aim in his mind – to tidy up the then current state of knowledge about useful Chinese medicinal herbs in Hong Kong. Through endless days of toil, he identified and investigated them, and eventually published his findings in a five-volume series of books with every plant illustrated in its natural surroundings in colour. Each one had its Chinese name, its known English name, and the equivalent Latin nomenclature checked by an expert traditional Chinese practitioner and a professor from the local Chinese University. The book, *Chinese Medicinal Herbs of Hong Kong*, was first printed in 1978 and then reprinted just two years later due to popular demand. It quickly became the essential textbook on herbal medicine for the thousands of traditional Chinese Medicine Practitioners working both locally and overseas. The book is his proud legacy, the culmination of his life-long dedication to Chinese medicinal herbs.

He was also fondly remembered as an enthusiastic scholar and teacher by his students in the Sun Yat Sen University in Kwang Zhou and by all of Hong Kong's traditional Chinese medicine practitioners. He was an energetic medical superintendent at the largest charity hospital in Hong Kong, as well as a caring head of the family, even though he never seemed to have enough time to spend with his children due to his busy schedule and all the wartime chaos that invariably upset everyone and everything. However, to be fair to him, when we were older, for a number of years post-WWII, he encouraged us to accompany him regularly on Sunday afternoons when he would go to the countryside, the hills and mountains, to enjoy hiking, bushwalking and herb-collecting excursions. That was something we always looked forward to. While on the trip, he would become very animated as he taught us about the herbs, so our hikes were always highly interesting.

The plant kingdom is fascinating. In it, we find the giant Californian bristlecone pine which has an unbelievable lifespan of over 5000 years. Just recently on a BBC documentary, the world's top naturalist Sir David Attenborough stood in front of a huge Californian Redwood, marvelling at the one-hundred-metre-tall giant specimen. And growing in the Eastern region of Australia, we have what is said to be the most poisonous tree on earth, called the gympie-gympie. The poison from its leaves is comparable to the venom from a scorpion or a funnel-web spider. The poison has not been fully assessed as yet, but it is suspected to be a small protein molecule that, if it penetrates your skin, somehow alters your nerve's sense of pain to an extreme degree so it feels like being burned by fire or acid. Even standing close to the tree can upset your system, making you unwell or even bleed from the nose. Yet beetles, birds and some kangaroos enjoy chewing the leaves!

But to return to the subject of metformin: it was used as a medicinal herb for decades until about 1957 when Sterne and his team discovered that metformin is a surprisingly effective remedy for NIDDM – and a very cheap one too. In most countries in the world, NIDDM sufferers are able to be afford the tablets as they are only a few cents each. The medication has very few side effects and is so safe that it can be bought over the counter without the need for a prescription in many countries such as Hong Kong and Thailand.

But recently – another surprise – metformin has been discovered to display many beneficial effects. Firstly, it mimics caloric restriction and activates SIRT I, in a way behaving like rapamycin, but not as a TOR inhibitor that suppresses rapamycin. In other words, it is capable of prolonging your lifespan, particularly if you can carry out CR at the same time – the combination is synergistic.

Secondly, metformin activates AMPK, another longevity regulator, which can restore the function of the energy-producing mitochondria, and produce more NAD (vitamin B3) to supply more fuel to sirtuins and activate other defences against ageing. It can inhibit cancer cells' metabolism, as reported in a study of forty-one thousand metformin users aged from sixty-eight to eighty-one. There are many other studies showing its effectiveness too. It is especially beneficial for the lungs, CRC and pancreas, and it reduces the risk of breast cancers by up to forty per cent.

So, metformin certainly appears to be an extremely safe substance, not only in medication for the treatment of NIDDM, but also used therapeutically to push back ageing and to help protect the body from cancer – all these wonderful benefits for a few pennies a day. What magic from the plant kingdom, and the awesome power of medicinal herbs!

AMPK

AMP-activated protein kinase (AMPK) is actually a metabolism-controlling enzyme, which has evolved to respond to low energy levels caused by taking metformin. Therefore, AMPK is used to restore mitochondrial function. Together with mTOR and sirtuins, AMPK has been regarded as one of the three main longevity pathways and can be activated by CR, exercise, and all of the wonder drugs previously mentioned, thereby enabling live organisms (including human beings) to become healthier, more resistant to disease, and longer living – our ultimate goal, without ever traveling overseas to look for the Fountain of Youth.

Chapter Six: Enter the Hi-tech Dragon

The modern hi-tech age

In this day and age, in the 2020s, we have to be grateful in Australia as we live in a peaceful, democratic country, distant from those zones where war, civil unrest, fighting and killing, bombing and murdering appear to be never ending daily occurrences. Yet, we are prepared to adopt climate change measures as set down in the Paris Agreement, in our realisation that extreme climate changes can cause uncontrollable bush fires (recall the disastrous one in 2020?) and severe drought, or damaging cyclones, torrential downpours and wide-spread flooding, all of which can and have resulted in lives lost and properties destroyed by the hundreds.

We are also fortunate in the sense that recently evolved knowledge and innovation in the tech space have provided us with numerous tools never before available. For example, just the invention of the computer and mobile phone have had an enormous global impact and changed our lives and behaviour forever – everywhere you go, by private car, by train, shopping, working in the office, travelling by air, you cannot do much without a computer being involved. They now come in all sorts of shapes and modules, and are capable of performing a wide range of functions based on specific programming. As we all know, rocket and space scientists would never have been able to send up a moon probe or the latest Mars explorer without computers and super computers that can perform tens of thousands of computations in less than a few seconds.

The rise of the mobile phone, or "smart phone", has been even more spectacular. Not long after its introduction, though it was initially a bulky gadget not much better than a WWII walkie-talkie, it was soon improved, and it has kept on improving rapidly so that, to my great surprise, when I was walking – or rather being pushed along – in Hong Kong's human current many years ago, everyone seemed to be chatting on a smart phone all the time – at the bus stop, on the pedestrian crossing, inside shops and hotels ... wherever and whenever.

It's no different in Sydney these days, although people appear more restrained and prefer to exercise their fingers – mainly their thumbs – and save their breath by texting or checking their emails whenever they have a chance to sit down on the train or on the platforms, hundreds of them, no one chatting because they have all fixed their gaze upon their smart phones. Recently you may notice some young males talking loudly to no one in particular while walking alone in the street or in a shopping centre, with two short white stalks sticking out from their ears, to give you a hint that they are using their Airpods.

When you sit down and ponder the matter, the smart phone is a genuinely hi-tech smart gadget evolved from our old-fashioned telephone set – you can communicate with your loved ones, family members and friends, or discuss business and problems, as long as you like, and from anywhere in the world, with whomever is on the address list on your phone. You can receive letters and notices, even contracts and agreements, from anyone, anytime via email and text message. You are even able to do banking, check your account or pay bills. All within seconds while having your morning coffee, and without bothering to get dressed to drive to the bank or the relevant government department, and without the bother of having to find a parking space and then join a queue.

Without the slightest doubt, these huge strides in high-tech innovation have saved us an enormous amount of time and inconvenience. Apps which enable you to download your favourite music and news have been available for a long time, while others let you count your steps or check your heartrate, not to mention the ubiquitous games. There are so many apps now that every individual can transform their device into their own personalised dream machine! You can even have a conversation with Siri if you want a chat.

The latest news today is that now school kids as young as seven are given 'wearables' which work like a mini-smart-phone-cum-watch, like Dick Tracy's fantastic watch in the old comic strip of many years ago. Like smart phones, they are getting cheaper and more affordable for many families, but that has increasingly become a thorny issue leading to much debate among school principals, teachers and parents.

Public transport

Since the first successful powered airplane flight in 1903 by American inventors Orville and William Wright, fast intercontinental air travel has become the norm because of the invention of the jet engine. The machine has rapidly advanced to be able to accommodate over five hundred passengers, many of these aeroplanes featuring twin decks and a wide body. These massive machines have been produced successfully on both sides of the world by companies such as Boeing in the US with its 747 jumbo jet, and the eponymous aircraft from the Airbus company in the EU. And, for a while, there was even the supersonic Concorde produced jointly by France and the UK. So, for years, jet planes have been everywhere, all over the world – inter-city and intercontinental, and these have been followed by budget, cut-price, competitive new-start airlines. Because of this, almost anyone can afford to travel by air, thereby saving time which equates to saving money.

Sadly, as the world witnessed, the coronavirus pandemic necessitated shutting down international borders from early 2020 with the aim of blocking viral transmission internationally and preventing even more deaths. As all flights were grounded, airports closed down globally and looked more like ghost towns than the busy bubbling transport centres they once were. Dozens of magnificent flying machines lay idle on the tarmac for more than a year, until the end of 2021.

However, many people just could not control their pent-up desire to travel as witnessed when the NSW-Victoria border restrictions dropped in late November 2020, and the Melbourne and Sydney airports suddenly came to life and were once more bustling with excited commuters milling around, happily pulling their luggage along to board their planes. The first batch of passengers arriving at Sydney were even met with all sorts of welcome banners and were treated like celebrities. And the equally excited CEO of Jetstar reported that flight numbers were up to fifty per cent of the normal, just on the first day.

Sadly, the bubble burst again, due to the relaxation of restrictions being premature as soon became obvious after recurring clusters of infected people began to surface intermittently, particularly in Victoria and NSW. We even witnessed ongoing intermittent interstate border shutdowns, often at short notice by alarmed state premiers. The imposition of restrictions produced a great deal of protest and frustration. And the prospect of smooth sailing is still a long way ahead again. People just must learn to be more patient, as mutations of Covid-19 appear. Only the successful mass vaccination of the world's population can provide more reassurance, and this has already begun in some countries, for example the free public vaccination started in the US by Joe Biden and in the UK by Boris Johnson. Australia, having fared better than most countries in the world, was slow to roll out the vaccinations and Sydney was therefore in a state of lockdown again for a good chunk of 2021.

Renewable energy

Of course, we cannot only concentrate on those measures which will allow us individually the best chance of a long life as none of us is isolated from our communities or the environment. If we are personally healthy but the planet is not, we will not get to enjoy our good health and long lives. We may avoid cancer and MI but that won't help us if the world becomes uninhabitable because of climate change or some other global catastrophe. So a discussion of the requirements of healthy aging and longevity would not be complete without some consideration of the measures we must take to ensure our own future, to say nothing of that of our children and grandchildren and all the other generations to come.

There are quite a few ways to produce energy without using fossil fuels like petrol, diesel, coal and wood. But the most practical and popular ones remain wind turbines, solar energy and hydroelectric power, which has been around the longest. These hi-tech solutions transform water, wind and solar energy into electricity without creating any dirty by-products like toxic gas and pollutants. The latest bright new idea has come from Elon Musk, the inventor and founder of the Tesla all-electric car, now officially proclaimed one of the world's richest men, who has invented "big batteries" that store up to one hundred and fifty megawatts of electricity. In fact, he has helped install over forty such big batteries all over Australia – and they work, particularly in South Australia where they dove-tail electricity supply from the batteries with the grid and reportedly saved the state from frequent breakdowns of the grid system and energy supply.

Clearly, Australia is appropriately named "the lucky country" for its sun-baked land covering a large area suitable for miles and miles of solar panels on farms. Its wide-open wind-swept coast stretching hundreds of miles forms an almost unlimited opportunity for the development of wind-turbine farms. We certainly have the means for Australia to reach its Paris agreement target of carbon-neutral status by 2050 or even earlier.

Developments in the area of environmentally friendly energy in Germany show what can be achieved. The Germans have designed and constructed about thirty thousand wind-turbine towers supplying nineteen per cent of the total energy supply (the second largest contribution to their power generation), outstripping coal and nuclear power. Each wind turbine is a hundred and seventy-nine metres high and capable of supporting five thousand homes.

The oldest renewable energy is from hydropower. China is currently leading the way with almost half of the thirty biggest hydroelectric power stations in the world. One of the most famous hydroelectric power plants outside of China is on the Niagara River, with its huge volume of water thundering down the horse-shoe shaped Niagara Falls and then a thirteen-kilometre stretch of waterfalls and rapids. The powerplant on the US side generates over two and a half million kilowatts, while the Canadian side has received two million kilowatts. And Australia has its own well known Snowy Mountain Hydroelectric Scheme, which is the largest engineering project ever undertaken in the nation. The plan for the pipeline is to invest a further three billion dollars in a renewal project that will revitalise hydroelectric power in Australia.

China, in addition to its Great Wall long famed as the world's biggest man-made structure, had started on its ambitions plan to store, control and put to good agricultural use the waters of its biggest and longest river, the Yangze River, along with its three gorges. They began building the world's largest dam structure in 1994 and completed it in 2006. The dam is two and a quarter kilometre long and must be very robust to withstand the tremendous water pressure generated during severe floods (and this has happened a few times in the last decades, not without a great deal of anxiety from supervising engineers).

Biogenetics

As Bill Gates stated in his book *The Road Ahead*, we needed a new way of thinking to give us the computer and the smart phone, in the same way that we needed innovative technology to give us the bullet train, the jumbo jet, the hybrid car, the electric motor car. By the same token, we now need new technology to provide us with renewable energy from wind turbines and solar panel, and we also need innovative ideas and the latest research and scientific thinking to explore the mystery of ageing, to make sure we can stop it advancing too fast and push it back, one step at a time.

So, this is what scientists do by performing numerous experiments on lab animals and fungus, based on the latest genetic and epigenetic findings. This sort of research has been going on for decades worldwide and has already provided many new discoveries, novel theories and proposed methodologies involving CR, exercise, lifestyle changes, and the currently available legal longevity drugs. All of these can be taken into consideration and implemented to make a start, but they need to be tailored to the individual rather than applied in a 'one-size-fits-all' approach.

Luckily some more good news has come to the fore regarding innovative procedures designed to resist the advance of ageing.

Protecting the telomere endcap

"Telomere" is a Greek term meaning end cap, and as we have seen already, it is basically a specific DNA-protein structure at both ends of each chromosome which protects it both from being disturbed and from excess attrition. Normally a telomere is eroded as a small portion is lost with every cell division. As the end cap wears out, the DNA strands become exposed and the molecule is flared and damaged until the cell is finished and becomes "senescent", meaning it has aged to the point of being worn until it is finally dead. Therefore, it is important to help the end cap maintain a healthy length by maintaining a lifestyle based around a healthy diet and regular exercise and the avoidance of smoking, addictive drugs and excessive alcohol use, as explained in Chapter Five.

What to do with senescent cells?

Our cells normally grow and divide and continue to function until there are breakages in the DNA strands due to many factors. The damage usually comes from the external environment, such as from radiation, whether it be from natural solar or artificial sun-tanning, CT scans or from unhealthy habits like smoking and drug taking. It may even occur due to viral infection. But generally, your cell's longevity genes – sirtuins – will have no trouble rushing to the site of damage to do the repairs. Then all returns to normal, and the cell continues to grow and divide as before.

However, when the damage is severe, like in a double-strand break, or with multiple breaks, or the telomere is worn completely thin, exposing the DNA protein, then the cell will treat all types of damage as a DNA break. It will stop dividing and become senescent if the damage is irreversible. As a senescent cell cannot divide to reproduce and is in a "zombie" state, it is still alive and can "panic" and discharge cytokines, causing inflammation all around it and upsetting both genome stability and the epigenome. This is damaging. So, senescence of cells is listed as one of the signs of ageing.

To eliminate this particular feature of ageing, we need to eliminate those senescent cells by killing them off. To do this we need to enlist the help of your immune system. Another alternative is to introduce a novelty "senolytic" drug which can target those zombie cells and digest them or recycle them. A trial on lab mice with two chemicals – quercetin and dasatinib – by J Kirkland at the Mayo clinic appeared to do just this. The lifespan of the treated mice was extended by thirty-six per cent.

A human trial was said to have been started in 2018, but if this is true the results have not yet been made public. But before we get too excited and start imagining people living to one hundred and forty or more, we have to be a bit more patient, and allow more experiments to be done to make sure similar beneficial results apply equally to humans, and to ascertain that there are no unacceptable side effects and long-term consequences from any form of new drugs. That said, this is a novel idea and brilliant minds are needed to lead the charge toward fresh developments. The prospects look pretty pink, if not yet rosy, because a senolytic drug, if all goes well, will no doubt reverse your age for a good time at least and you will feel younger, have more energy and experience less disease and disability.

Cloning

In 1996, Ian Wilmut and his colleagues at the University of Edinburgh replaced the chromosome of a sheep's egg with those from an udder cell and out came a new sheep, "Dolly", a clone. She lived only half as long as a normal sheep but only because it caught a lung disease. The significance for our subject is that it showed chromosomes from an ageing animal still retain all digital information, and this can be passed onto a young clone to create a younger version of the original.

Cloning has since been carried out successfully on many other animals including dogs and cows. It is now routinely done to produce better farm animals and racehorses. And behind these experiments' profound effects is the near-magical concept that ageing can be reset, probably even in humans, though there would be a great deal of controversy, resistance and legal battles in various sectors of society due to ethical considerations which make this a social and legal minefield, at least for now.

Cellular reprogramming

Shinya Yamanata, a Japanese stem-cell specialist and researcher, discovered that a combination of four genes (Oct4, Klf4, Sox2, and c-Myc) could transform adult cells into stem cells which, being multi-potent and immature, can be turned into any form of cell tissue because they can be coded for the powerful transcription factors that control all other genes in development. This means they have the ability to copy genetic information onto a strand of RNA. For this incredible discovery, he won the Nobel prize in 2012.

These four genes, now called *Yamanata factors*, are regarded as leading us to two new directions. Firstly, they can be used in the lab to grow entirely new cells, tissue and even organs to give patients in need a new lease of life. With a kidney transplant, for example, someone suffering renal failure could have their life extended by at least a few more years, if not decades. Secondly, the Yamanata factors look like being one of the switches to reset not only worn-out or aged organs, but possibly an entire body! And once "reset" you will feel ten or twenty years younger – no more grey hair, no more flabby and wrinkled skin, and far more energy… fancy being transformed like that. The whole concept sounds out of this world. But based on recent biogenetic discoveries and hundreds of animal experiments, it could be done, at least in theory.

The concept is not too far from "gene therapy", but the procedure needs to be explored further experimentally and there needs to be more scientific discussion to evaluate its viability. It is important for us to wait to ensure there wouldn't be any serious mishaps, complications and damage to the human body, or any functional disturbance of any organs. The procedure would appear to run like this: the four Yamanata factors would be injected into the body as "reprogramming" genes, or as a switch, so to speak. As mentioned, they can induce adult cells to become stem cells which are pleuro-potent and able to replace ageing cells and organs later on when given further direction or provided with some activating trigger.

Without this, they are likely to stay dormant after they are injected into the subject, ideally when they are about forty years old and in the vicinity of the onset of ageing. By then their immune system and most organs are starting to wear out and they are feeling run down after decades of work and worries. Their body would now be storing a good supply of Yamanata genes but they would not feel any effects, nevermind feeling younger, until they took a steady dose of some chemicals to activate those genes (or, shall we say, to flick the switch on). Some sort of common antibiotic such as doxycycline (a harmless broad spectrum antibiotic) seems to be an appropriate choice. And chemicals like rapamycin seem to possess a magical molecular structure that can work like a special enzyme to activate this process. Even vitamin C has been mentioned as a potential trigger. My impression is that these small chemicals, enzymes, amino acids and proteins, like sirtuins, catalase and MNR, can get in and out of the cell and participate in hundreds of intracellular reactions, or co-ordinate numerous chemical reactions in the body. But a great deal more work and experimentation in this area is required to convince the world.

You probably would not feel young immediately, but perhaps soon thereafter, when the stem cells have commenced working to refresh and reorganise your organs and immune system and rejuvenate your whole body. It will take time but the transformation will progress steadily until you begin to look and feel younger, both internally and externally; perhaps ten, maybe twenty years younger, depending on the type of genes put in, and the correct dose.

The four Yamanata factors need to be used with caution. They are said to be quite toxic if administered in too high a dose and can give the recipient teratoma, which is a mixed mass of various tumours or tissues possibly derived from some remnants of multi-potent embryonic cells like stem cells. To minimise such a mishap, researchers may prefer to use only three of the four Yamanata factors which would still have a powerful but beneficial effect.

Vaccines

Vaccines, vaccines and more vaccines! Mention vaccines, and it arouses a mixed feeling in many people. I am sure that by now everyone – from wealthy people in the developed world to poverty-stricken refugees in improvised camps – will never be able to erase it from their memories because of the panic caused by the coronavirus pandemic. The virus swept through the world infecting two hundred and five nations and territories on its first wave, and again a hundred and twenty nations on its second wave. By November 2020, over forty-five million people had tested positive for the virus, and over one million had died. The scene in the US in particular was disheartening with the incumbent president Donald Trump taking a "couldn't be bothered" attitude while putting all his energy into winning votes for a second term as president. He totally ignored the wise advice from his chief medical officer Dr Fauci and all warnings and rules from the WHO. Even his National Security Adviser John Bolton (who had served three past presidents) resigned after spending many of his four hundred and fifty three White House days with Trump, due to his frustration and realisation that Trump was "addicted to chaos, deeply suspicious of his government and showing a lot of bizarre behaviour". He tried to talk his way out of the public health crisis – a real serious matter for the country – yet only ended up undercutting his own and the nation's credibility. He shocked many nations by disengaging from the WHO, and cutting off funding to the organisation. It was frightening to see the reported death rate rising spectacularly high and fast, reaching over three thousand persons a day, almost every day for months on end. Brazil and India were also catching up fast. Only six high profile nations emerged as winners – Australia, New Zealand, Singapore, South Korea, Taiwan and Japan. As 2022 progresses, each country has had its ups and downs but total deaths over the course of the pandemic still remain below one hundred and fifty per million, with New Zealand having less than fifteen per million! This is very low when we consider that deaths in the twenty-four hardest hit nations rose at times to above two thousand five hundred deaths per million inhabitants, and in some countries double that number.

There was much news of research work and trial testing of Covid-19 vaccines by research institutions, pharmaceutical companies and university labs in many countries, all seemingly fighting to be the first to produce an effective vaccine with the least side effects. But few ordinary people outside the vaccine research world are knowledgeable in regard to the difficulties involved in producing a brand-new vaccine, as the process involves many steps. First, scientists must obtain the virus DNA or amino acid and then allow the suitable messenger RNA to contact the virus surface, particularly the "spikes" so characteristic of Covid-19. Once that has been done, immune cells (the T-cells from the bone marrow and the thymus) get re-educated on how to recognise the "marked" virus and block the attack by picking them up and eliminating them. Following this, a prolonged period is required to trial test the vaccine – firstly on lab animals, then a further three trials on humans, and a subsequent follow-up period involving more testing and checking to make sure that the new vaccine is really safe and effective on humans. This means that the an antibody found to be able to kill the coronavirus can actually be produced by the host's immune system. In the meantime, the test subject must be checked repeatedly for a longer period to rule out any side effects.

One critical concept we must keep in mind is that with any infection, the individual's immune system will usually have a huge impact on their chances of survival. Out of the more than four hundred million Covid-19 positive cases, as of February 2022, over three hundred million have recovered, mostly due to their superior immune system, while close to six million have perished, the majority of whom are elderly people with co-morbidities like NIDDM, CVD and Alzheimers, meaning they have a very weakened immunity. This is why so many deaths have occurred in nursing homes and retirement villages.

Not many young healthy people died from the infection, except perhaps those leading unhealthy lifestyles, or already suffering respiratory system problems like asthma. Then there are those who ignore the advice from the health authorities, unable to distinguish fake news and bogus science from good authoritative counsel. As a result, we have the high profile but controversial actions of demonstrators who resist such sensible measures as wearing masks, taking vaccines and observing lockdowns.

Throughout the course of the pandemic, it has been clear that children usually recover quickly, pre-emptively we might say, due to the swift response of their immune system, as if they had already been immunised against Covid-19. My experience in general practice makes this no surprise, and anyone who observes children inside and outside their schools will almost always find they are physically very active, running around in school yards chasing each other, yelling and screaming. In other words, with their high basal metabolic rate and regular good exercise, their vitality genes are strong, vigorous and protect them from epidemic virus infections in general. All the more reason to ensure that they don't spend too much time watching TV, playing video games or on their phones.

So normally it would take a few years for a new and reliable vaccine to complete safety requirements and receive official approval from the local regulatory body (this is how, for instance, the historic smallpox and the polio vaccines were created). Only then are they allowed to be used on the general population. Now Australian readers might say "what about the flu vaccine that we get every year? How come we get the shot every year on time before the flu season?" They would be quite correct to point this out.

The difference is that as the flu virus mutates almost every year and usually starts in the Northern Hemisphere, our vaccine supplier the CSL (Commonwealth Serum Lab) is usually able to obtain the prevalent strain or strains of the flu virus, identify their DNA configuration and manufacture the flu vaccine in time before the flu season. As the CSL has been meeting this challenge year after year, it has understandably become quite proficient at this, so the production of the flu vaccine is usually simpler and quicker than it would be if the virus was a brand new and complex strain.

After a great deal of controversy over the competing vaccines, three were rolled out. One in the US from Pfizer, which claimed that its vaccine was about ninety per cent effective after three test trials. But the vaccine needs to be stored at below seventeen degrees Celsius at all times until a week before vaccination – a rather inconvenient storage method, and not practical for many developing nations. The second one produced by Moderna claims to be almost ninety-five per cent effective and does not require deep freeze storage. Number three is Oxford-Astra Zeneca from the UK, who also announced that their vaccine is seventy to ninety per cent effective. It was rushed through the approval process by the PM Boris Johnson and the UK health authority in order to start mass vaccination in December 2020 due to the seriously urgent Covid-19 situation in that nation. Both the US and Australia were not far behind either.

In early 2021, Johnson & Johnson in the US claimed to have developed their own brand of Covid-19 vaccine which required only one shot to get up to 66.3 percent protection. It sounds convenient, but is not recommended as a primary nor secondary vaccine due to its reported serious side-effect of blood clotting. Even if used as a first dose, it is recommended to have a secondary vaccine of either Pfizer or Moderna within two months.

Outside the Western countries, Russia had claimed to have already produced their own Covid-19 vaccine, and started mass vaccinations beginning with President Putin's daughter to show how confident they were about the safety of their brand of vaccine. Despite early controversy over the quick release of the drug prior to stage three testing, it has been widely used and the evidence has mounted as to its safety and efficiency. At about the same time, China also made it known to the world that they had produced their own brand of vaccine and they then initiated their own mass vaccination programme, and sent millions of free doses to some friendly SEA countries. This vaccine was the first produced outside the West approved by the WHO. To date there has been no report of untoward side effects.

Australia's own roll-out of the vaccine was far from optimal. After a blood clot scare with, it was decided that those below fifty years old should wait for the Pfizer type while the front-line workers, anyone over fifty and those with medical conditions would get still be given Astra Zeneca. This was met with some consternation, especially by the elderly who felt that they were being given an inferior product with a greater chance of side effects.

The dramas with the vaccine are not yet over as the effectiveness of vaccination over time has been questioned, with it seeming that Pfizer is more prone to losing its potency quickly than AstraZeneca. As of mid-2022, it has been recommended that a fourth shot and possibly a periodic one after that will be required to keep people safe. Also, the virus has already mutated a number of times, so it is clear there is no room for complacency.

Nonetheless, Covid-19 vaccines will play a crucial role in increasing longevity as the vaccinated public will recover their health and be able to stick to a healthy lifestyle to keep pushing against ageing. So we all must proceed with vaccination, as advised by medical experts, and ignore the fake news and ignorant propaganda from anti-vaxxers and other clusters of people with warped vested interests, both in Australia and overseas. While the side effects that these people rave about are real, they are usually quite mild, like a weak dose of flu, and you may be wise to take a day off to help protect your immune system and avoid strenuous exercise for a few days.

Genetic scanning (DNA scanning)

To return to the topic of human genes and the genome: the human body has about three trillion cells, and each cell has in its nucleus twenty-three pairs of chromosomes. Each one of the chromosomes is a compact structure of twin DNA strands twisted around each other – the famous double helix which is composed of 3.234 billion base pairs of amino acids, referred to as "letters". This sequence is called "the genetic code". DNA has all the genetic information of an organism encoded in digital form.

Not that long ago, we tended to look at the intriguing, complex structure of DNA with an awe which could be overwhelming, particularly if we looked at the double helix on a screen in some computerised representation, turning round and round – it certainly impressed on us what a marvel of nature it is. But in 1990, the Human Genome Project was launched. It lasted ten years at a cost a few billion US dollars for a single gene. This was a huge achievement given the technology of the time, and it has been applauded as a milestone in biogenetic history. Later, when it first became possible to have your own genetic scan done by a bio-tech lab in the US, the cost was phenomenal.

Nowadays, according to Professor Sinclair, the entire human genome of twenty-five thousand genes can be scanned in only a few days for under a hundred dollars. And all he has to do is to plug a DNA sequencer into a laptop to get the result; how amazing the strides made in technology have been in the last thirty years!

Genetic scanning can be lifesaving, as shown in a real case reported in the *Sydney Morning Herald* in October 2020. Apparently, a healthy young Australian rower, an Olympic hopeful, with no past diseases of note, was doing routine training on a rowing machine in one of the training centres in Italy. When he had finished his training, he got up from the machine and collapsed on the floor. Had this collapse happened when he was rowing in the water, he may have drowned and died.

Fortunately, by a bit of luck, the in-house coach or trainer not only performed a successful resuscitation, but also sent him for a genetic scan. It revealed that this young man had a hidden faulty gene called the "cardiac arrest gene", which meant that his heart could suddenly stop beating without any reason if that rogue gene played up. This discovery effectively destroyed his hopes of training for the Olympics, but at the same time, it has literally saved his life, even though moving forward he needed a regular heart check by a cardiologist to forestall future attacks and was only allowed to do gentle exercise like walking. So the value of this kind of clinical testing cannot be under-estimated and should be, like cardiac defibrillators, freely and widely available in hospitals and clinics once the cost has become more affordable.

DNA testing has lately been applied in wider fields to be included not only as a means of making the early diagnosis of a disease, genetic or hereditary, but also to detect the genetic signatures of cancers and tumours way before they are normally perceivable, and long before they turn malignant. Our cells can become damaged and turn abnormal and pre-cancerous for various reasons. One of the most trendy and popular concepts from past decades has been the theory of "oxidative stress" caused by cellular DNA and mitochondria being under incessant bombardment by oxidants during the cellular metabolic process. But this theory has already been found to lack sufficient convincing evidence, as mentioned in Chapter Four.

So nowadays most scientists regard DNA damage and cellular changes as being quite often due to exposure to chemicals (carcinogens and pre-carcinogens) from cigarette smoking, chemical sprays (domestic or agricultural or industrial) and radiation (solar, X-ray machine or CT scan). The younger immature cells, like young, undifferentiated blood cells and stem cells in particular, can have their DNA badly damaged, and as a result begin behaving differently. Under the microscope, cancer cells show up on tests as a darker blue, they have a bigger nucleus and grow in a more disorderly fashion. Abnormal protein fragments may detach or discharge from the surface of those cells, entering into the bloodstream where they can be detected by a lab blood test. The results of the test can be combined with the data from a genetic DNA test to allow the clinician to make a more definitive diagnosis and recommend the most appropriate therapy.

Some pre-malignant cells, like those in the prostate, may discharge an increasing amount of protein or chemical (the PSA – prostate specific antigen), an early sign of cancer developing, which means it is growing abnormally larger and is labelled "hyperplastic". This serves as a warning sign for the patient's doctor to keep a closer eye on his progress.

This is a new and exciting development has been made possible because the mapping of the human genome has been completed, new hi-tech gadgets like DNA sequencers are available, and there are intense ongoing scientific studies focusing on our subcellular level. The powerful currents of knowledge flowing from many scientific centres and institutes have become the prime mover in achieving what we are witnessing today, resulting in novel diagnostics and treatments. These developments apply not only to chronic diseases and cancers; they are also helping us to open the hitherto locked door of ageing by enlightening us as to its causes, and putting us on the path to discover how to slow down its advance.

This sort of DNA scanning could possibly be developed further, so it is available in a device not unlike our smart phone. Such a development would enable us to perform proactive personal scanning with a home scanner, or even a wearable wristwatch-type device which continuously monitors our body.

New Organs for Old

These days, the most common orthopaedic surgery is none other than 'replacement' of hip joints and knee joints with an artificial one made from a combination of metal and plastic. If your kidneys are damaged by disease, or inflamed, or have some congenital defects to the stage that you need to consider replacing them with new ones from donation from a live person or someone recently deceased (the victim of a motor vehicle accident, for instance). It has also been proposed that "xenotransplantation" may become a viable option. This is the transplantation of a genetically modified organ from another species, specially bred pigs being the favoured alternative to date. This is currently the most promising solution to the dearth of human organs available. However, this technology has not yet been perfected. There are three main problems to overcome:

The pig has to be specially bred and genetically modified by knocking out the alpha-1.3 galactosyltransferase gene which is responsible for hyperactive rejection of the transplant.

Some special genes have to be introduced in the human recipient to help their body to accept the pig's organ.

The xenotransplantation procedure has to be presented to the FDA for approval.

So far, two cases of pig-to-human kidney xenotransplantation to two brain-dead human recipients have been reported on the prestigious NEJM and reported as successful when both kidneys were observed functioning normal with even improved eGFR.

Recently an American by the name of David Bennett, who was fifty-seven years old with a badly failing heart, received the first ever xenotransplantation from a genetically modified pig heart on 7 January 2022. The news was well-publicised all over the world. The operation was performed at the Maryland Hospital as a last-ditch experiment because the patient had no other options.

Bennett appeared to be recovering during the two months post-op until he started to deteriorate rapidly and died. The most likely cause of death was considered to be a hyperacute rejection, infection and other cardiac complications.

So for the moment this is not a viable option. So if your heart has gone into failure and you need a new one – you may need a regular heart transplant. Heart transplants in Australia has had an exciting history though it includes the tragic end of the legendary heart surgeon Dr Victor Chang.

Victor Chang was a fellow alumnus of mine from St Paul's high school which we attended in Hong Kong. He was sent to Sydney University in 1951 and graduated from there in 1962 with First Class Honours. He was then sent to the UK to receive more training in surgery under a cardiac surgeon after which he spent two more years training at the Mayo Clinic. After his return to St Vincent's Hospital in Sydney, he worked with Harry Windsor, the cardiac surgeon who performed Australia's first heart transplant.

Around 1980, as better anti-rejection drugs were used with success, Victor Chang was able to lobby politicians and businessmen to establish a heart-transplant programme at the SVH. Then in 1984, he and his team made the headlines when they successfully performed a heart transplant on Fiona Coote, aged fourteen, the youngest transplant patient at that time. From 1984 – 1990, his team performed one hundred and ninety-seven heart and fourteen heart-lung transplants with the phenomenal success rate of ninety per cent. For all his service and contribution to cardiac surgery and society, Chang was awarded an AC (Companion of the Order of Australia) in 1986.

From that time on, he led research in the development of an artificial heart, and organised production of inexpensive heart valves for his patients in SEA.

Tragedy struck on 4 July 1991 in a failed extortion attempt in the Sydney suburb of Mosman, when two greedy, and clearly inexperienced thugs from Malaysia – Liew and Lim rammed Chang's car and demanded money (originally they had intended to kidnap Chang for ransom). When Chang refused, one of the thugs shot him twice in the head and ran away, but the murderer was caught and put in prison for twenty to twenty-six years. The criminals were subsequently deported to Kuala Lumper after parole.

Victor was not only a brilliant cardiac surgeon, he was innovative and very caring toward his patients. He left quite a legacy in Sydney, and has been commemorated with a life-size bronze statue situated at the Victor Chang Cardiac Research Institute which was launched in 1994 by the then prime minister Paul Keating under the patronage of Kerry Packer. Victor himself had set up a Victor Chang Foundation for the education and research into cardiology and cardiothoracic surgery. In 1999, the then prime minister, John Howard (another graduate of Sydney University), honoured Victor Chang as the Australian of the Century. In 2017, even one of the Sydney icon ferries was named after him.

I had the honour of meeting Victor years ago when I was a member of Melbourne's Australian Chinese Medical Association which invited him to give a talk on some cardiac surgery procedures. It was a great inspiration for our members, some of whom were either his contemporaries or fellow alumni. He even showed our members a video on how he performed a heart-surgery procedure while talking gently and clearly to his team and enthusiastic student audience during the operation.

Victor Chang impressed everyone as a brilliant and innovative cardiac surgeon, who not only cared about his patients, but also acted as an inspirational role model for the younger generation of aspiring cardiac surgeons.

Nowadays any failed organ can be replaced, except the brain – which is most unfortunate when we consider the life story of the famed and popular neurosurgeon, Chris O'Brien. He was one of the most popular and beloved Australian head and neck cancer surgeons, who in a cruel twist of fate, was discovered to have an aggressive and lethal brain cancer in 2006. Despite the fact that this cancer is generally lethal, he had the courage to go through four operations on his brain conducted by Charles Teo, another brilliant neurosurgeon. With his stoic slogan of 'Never say Die' which became the title of his book, he pulled through and went on his crusade to set up the Sydney Cancer Centre, with the sympathetic backing of Kevin Rudd, the prime minister at the time, who assisted with the funding. O'Brien's life story is a sterling example of how strong faith, great courage and unfading willpower can help an individual to overcome immense adversity.

A new approach to solving body part and rejection problems may be the new technology of 3-D printing. The principle is to obtain body organ cells or tissue from the intended recipient and grow them. This material will then be used in a 3-D printer to suite the blueprint of your organ which serves as the template. The cells based on your own and generated in the laboratory will be fed into the printer, which will built them up layer by layer until they have printed a new organ almost identical to your own but without the defects. The new organ can then be transplanted in situ and replace the diseased or worn out one. One of the main differences from normal 3-D computer printing is that the material used is biocompatible plastic.

This is not a fantasy anymore – it has been successfully done both in Australia and overseas, though at the moment mostly for basic tissues, occasionally even mini-organs. For example, in 2018, the University of Newcastle made the first 3D-printed human cornea.

One of the main troubles with the3-D printing of human organs is that the organ would collapse because the cavity structure (for example the heart). So the scientists nowadays experiment two new ways to pop up the products by 1) suspending it in hydrogel serving as scaffolding, 2) to print the organ while in outer space relying on the weightlessness. In fact, the experiment in orbit was started in 2019 and upgraded in 2021.

At this stage, however, those pioneering researchers admit that even though 3-D printing of human organs is practicable, it is not easy to recreate the full function of the transplanted organ, and it may need another ten to fifteen years for printed organs to be fully functional. Or, as mentioned before, take your own stem cells and direct them to form the desired organ, as explained in the section on Yamanata factors.

With all this human ingenuity and technological advance there are many exciting avenues for researchers and scientists to explore and develop. As new technologies emerge and are perfected until they are safe and legal, people will find themselves with an increasing number of resources to access in the fight to turn the tide on aging.

Chapter Seven: Wonders of the Green World

Fabulous Foods – Nutrients and Energy

The Chinese, like most people with common-sense, have long recognised that food is the very foundation of life. Over two thousand years ago, that most revered teacher and philosopher, Confucius, declared to his disciples that "food and sex are human nature and instinct", not that anyone who loves eating, loves sex, and loves good food needs a philosopher to argue the case for them.

Chinese cuisine has been named the best in the world, the most elaborate, the most magnificently presentable and the tastiest, and this is not without reason. There are many factors behind the success story of Chinese cuisines. Firstly, Chinese cuisine is prepared in up to thirty or forty different ways. By comparison Western cooking, including world-class French and Italian cuisines utilises only eight or nine methods. I have not reinstated these comments because not only are they irrelevant to your general subject they are irrelevant to your sub-subject here which is Chinese cooking. It doesn't fit the context at all. The Chinese chef chooses how to cook according to the type of meats, the greens, the ingredients including the spices, and adjusts the timing to cook them until they are just tender and not over-cooked. This is especially important for expensive seafoods like lobsters, scallops, sea-urchins, etc.

Secondly, chefs usually learn their trade through apprenticeship, helping the head chef and observing what they are doing. It may need quite a few years of practice to be able to turn out magnificent dishes like those nine-course or sometimes eleven-course banquet cuisines which are served on important occasions. But those well-motivated young chefs work hard, train hard, and spend long hours honing to perfect their skills.

Thirdly, with several thousand years' experience with cooking, the Chinese have just about experimented with cooking almost everything edible, including fungus, black or white, reptiles, insects and fowl, sea creatures like sea urchins, sea cucumbers, jellyfish, and all sorts of animals, including dogs and cats ... in short 'anything that moves'.

It may sound unusual or cruel, depending on one's culture or personality, but during its 5000 years of history, China has gone through quite a few natural disasters and major upheavals including famines and catastrophic droughts, floods and civil wars. So the farmers and villagers have had to do their best to survive on whatever they could salvage from the fields, the forest, and the rivers, including their own pets, and, when in crisis situations, even tree roots and bark. It should be remembered that survival is the most basic instinct and many people have even resorted to cannibalism in extreme circumstances, regardless of their usual cultural norms. Here we are ignoring the fact that in some cultures, historically, rather than being taboo, cannibalism was considered a sacred act.

While it is obvious that everyone must eat to live, currently the Chinese (particularly the Cantonese) are fond of a different sentiment where dining is concerned. They like to say 'we live to eat'! This is because, as every Chinese person knows, Canton city (the capital of Kwang Tung province), has long been famous for its super-cuisines and is nick-named the 'gourmet food' city where exquisite dinners of nine to twelve courses are commonplace for the locals.

In order to fight off chronic disease and push back ageing, we still eat every day to build up our energy and nourish our longevity genes. Generally we do this three times a day, unless we are practising 'intermittent fasting'. Food is nourishment and eating good food is not only a pleasant indulgence, but it can also act as tasty medicine that helps your immune system to fight off diseases.

But, before we start to shop and buy foods for cooking, we will go through the most important concept of how food is classified. Basically, every food can be categorised as either a macro- or micro-nutrient.

Macronutrients

Under this heading are the most important foods – the carbohydrates (carbs), fats and oils (fatty acids) and proteins.

Carbohydrates

When carbs, like rice and bread, become broken down and digested in our intestines to become the basic unit of glucose molecules, the glucose passes through the intestinal wall, into the bloodstream where it is distributed to all of the cells in the body. These absorb the metabolic ingredients and turn them into energy. This is the famous Krebs cycle which occurs in mitochondria. Alternately energy is produced in the form of a more complex molecule called glycogen, which is created by enzymes in the cell and sent to the liver for storage.

Carbs come from all sorts of grains and cereals, the most simple ones being ordinary sugars from sugar canes and beetroots and honey, as well as vegetables, especially the stems and root vegetables like sweet potatoes. All kind of fruits and legumes, from peas to peanuts also contain carbohydrates. Glucose in fact is the main food for energy for our whole body, and your brain depends entirely on glucose for its energy and function. That is why carbs should compose the bulk of your daily food for your instant energy needs because your body's cells are extremely efficient in tuning sugar into heat and energy with no complicated metabolites. And your body needs energy to function normally all the time.

But please note here that we recommend that you consume those whole grain, unrefined and unprocessed carbs, such as brown rice or basmati brown rice, rather than that well-polished, beautiful white rice. Barley is also excellent (unhulled rather than the pearl variety), rolled oats for porridge, corn – a rather sweet kernel studded cob. Rye is also recommended in bread and should preferably be sourdough.

All of the above unprocessed cereals are loaded with good proteins, minerals, vitamins and polyphenols, making up to from thirty per cent to three hundred per cent of the recommended daily allowance for your bodily needs, but much of the nutritional content could be lost through processing when grains are 'whitened' and 'polished'.

As always, find the organic variety, even though it may cost a fraction more and require somewhat longer cooking time, but it will provide your body with more nutrients than the non-organic type.

Lipids, Oils, Fats

When ingested, lipids or oils break down into simple fatty acids. There are up to at least forty different kind of fatty acids classed as non-essential fatty acids (NEFA) which will be burnt off as fuel by your body. These produce more sustained energy, twice as much heat and energy, in fact, as carbs produce. But the body retains the omega 3 and omega 6 oils for the production of important hormones and enzymes. Omega 3 comes from fish, and omega 6 from plants, and both are classified as good oils.

Omega 3 helps fish to be mobile and flexible in very cold water in the deep sea. This is why it is effective in cleaning cholesterol out our arteries. Under similar conditions, saturated oils and bad oils like margarine, butter and lard would all turn solid (like they do in your own fridge). This is why they block up the arteries.

Proteins

These are the most important form of macronutrient in so far as they form the basic building blocks for our bodies. Proteins occur in animals as well as in the plant kingdom. Humans generally ingest protein in the form of meat sourced from land animals, fowls and sea animals, as well as all kinds of plants and legumes.

All proteins are broken down in our digestive tract into basic amino acids (the simplest type) and peptides (the more complex forms) before they are absorbed thru the gut wall and then into the blood where twenty or more varieties of amino acids may be found at a time. Nine of the essential amino acids are not found in any plants except soya beans.

All these amino acids will be absorbed by the cells and combined into important proteins, hormones and enzymes which will be used for a variety of purposes. For example, the thyroid gland needs them to form thyroglobulins (hormones used to control the body's metabolic rate); the skeletal system needs them to form scaffolding for calcium mineral absorption which builds strength and allows developing bodies to grow taller; and every single one of our three trillion cells need amino acids to repair DNA, cell membranes, and all of the parts of the body that need their protein components regularly replaced. Each of our DNA helixes has almost three and a quarter billion base pairs of amino acids arranged in a set sequence. So during cell division and growth, which are natural perpetual ongoing cellular activities, lots of amino acids are required at all times.

So proteins should be the last nutrients to be burned as fuel while carbs and oils are better utilised as fuel to supply energy to your whole body. Nowadays, you must keep very cool and alert about the bewildering number of choices urged upon you in the form of 'new' diets, new medicines or gadgets. These unproven gimmicks present in all forms of media and social media are continually bombarding us and challenging your intelligence. They often claim to be 'scientifically proven' or 'approved' but, in fact, are not backed by reputable medical experts or valid research, and are mostly promoted by snake-oil salesman and 'get rich quick' new start-ups. It is wisest to treat them the same as you would 'fake news' and unsolicited mobile phone calls. Stick to the basic well-established principles of nutrition which take into account our body's normal function.

Micronutrients

In this group of chemicals we find vitamins and some minerals. We don't normally need to ingest much of any one of these, maybe less than one gram a day. They usually function as a catalyst or as enzymes which accelerate cellular reaction but they are not used up in the process.

Vitamins exist in one of two forms with A, D, E and K being fat soluble and vitamin C and the B group being water soluble. All of them are very important and are ignored at your peril. You may recall that vitamin B3, the precursor of Nicotinamide MN, is required in over five hundred intracellular reactions, and supplies fuel to sirtuins which enables them to work faster and helps them to rescue us from the advance of ageing.

Here, we must refresh our memory about Minerals, which are also classified as micronutrients, and are mainly found in our bodily fluids, blood, inside and outside of the cells as intra- and extra- cellular fluids which serve as a special medium which helps maintain optimal pH: 7.35 – 7.45, i.e. slightly alkaline. This creates the ideal environment for optimal enzyme reactions which also depend on body temperature to achieve their maximum speed and power – if you recall the reaction inside the cell is so fast and complex as to be beyond our imagination. For these complex and not-so-complex reactions we need common inorganic elements like sodium, chloride, potassium, calcium, sulphur and phosphorus to be in fairly correct concentrations. Normally we don't have to worry about them even if blood tests show minor differences from normal as based on the lab's manual This is because your kidneys play the role of regulating the level of micronutrients in your body twenty-four hours a day, three hundred and sixty-five days a year. they keep your blood and fluid pH finely tuned within that narrow range which keeps every organ humming happily.

Green Power (Phytonutrients)

Let's review what we have learned about longer lifespan from all previous chapters.

The earlier chapters about centenarians and super-centenarians and how they live, what they eat and the lifestyle they keep while setting a good example for their family and getting along in their community, should have left you with no doubt in your mind that the human lifespan has been proven to be able to reach one hundred years and beyond, even without any modern aids and medication. This vital new knowledge drawn from demographic studies which have been made possible by scientists and investigative journalists putting in a lot of hard work and research.

Then we saw how the mystery of why we age has been unravelled with the discovery of small chemicals or enzymes called sirtuines and STACs that are the longevity or the vitality genes. These greatly help push ageing back which is now regarded as a disease like High Blood pressure, diabetes or osteoarthritis that can be controlled or pushed back to enable us live longer.

But we also need many chemicals to activate the longevity genes to repair DNA damage, to turn genes on and off, to boost our immune system and to protect us against diseases. These chemicals are called Polyphenols, and Isofavonds, of which there are as many as several thousands. They are usually found in the plant kingdom, in the form of colourful vegetables, flowers and fruits. Most of them are still a mystery to us in regard to their formula, their effects on our system, and their interaction with our cellular metabolism. Some are already manufactured in tablet/capsule form as supplements, but it is advisable for you to eat as many whole vegies and as much fruit as often as you can, because supplements contain usually one or, at the most, two chemicals, while the plants contain many more nutrients and other polyphenols to help your system, according to much current scientific belief. Take the well-known Resveratrol which is an extract from red wine such as pinot noir and has been regarded as a key factor helping the French to protect their CVS by reducing their bad cholesterol which more or less explains the enigmatic phenomenon called the 'French Paradox'.

However, subsequent studies suggest that Resveratrol by itself may not confer the full benefit that drinking red wine does. This is because the wine has many other polyphenols in it. A bottle of red wine, by standard analysis, while it contains a mere 1-5 mg of Resveratrol, also contains 1-2 gm per litre of polyphenols and procyanidin: a proven powerful anti-oxidant. In other words, having a glass of good red is far better than buying supplements or drugs/medication from pharmacy.

The Power of the Plant Kingdom

Why are we so focussed on plants: colourful flowers, naturally fresh green leafy vegetables, beautifully tempting fruits? What have they got to do with our pursuit of the Fountain of the Youth? How do they function as secret weapons to fight cancers, tumours and all those common diseases like heart attacks, asthma, chronic diseases like NIDDM, osteoarthritis, and the mysterious Alzheimer's disease?

Well, the plant kingdom has had enormous power to keep humans (and all other living animals) alive and healthy ever since we first emerge on this earth three million years ago. For practical purposes, what we eat every day should be mostly sourced from the plant kingdom – rice, wheat, oats and other grains; we have constantly emphasised that we need to have at least one third of potion of vegies and fruit, and a minimum of meat on our plates. And in the end meat itself derives from the grass and fodder the animals we eat are raised on. All healthy diets will have three vegies and five fruits if possible, as is clearly illustrated on any genuine food pyramid you might see in a pharmacy or dietitian's and nutritionist's offices.

When you are sick, some of the medications prescribed by your GP could contain drugs derived from plants, since the twenty-five per cent of prescription drugs are sourced this way. And the cup of tea or coffee or chocolate and fruit drinks are all made from plants and usually reasonably cheap except during a poor harvest. For example, it has been reported recently that vanilla has gone up sky-high in price due to a poor harvest for the last three years as the crops on Madagascar (which producing two thirds of the world's supply) have been wiped out by cyclones. So your ice cream isn't vanilla now because the vanilla beans are as expensive as silver – $8 for one bean, just one bean, not one kilogram! – it is just simple logic that vanilla is no longer affordable for the average person.

Green plants are our lifesavers. They give us fuel and energy to move our body parts, keep our hearts beating, or lung working, and our more than three trillion cells thriving and growing. And now some of those Polyphenols and Flavonoids from plants can activate our longevity genes to repair damaged DNA, to switch on good genes or silence bad ones. Such wonderful co-operation could not happen without those ingenious chemicals from the plant kingdom, or from the miraculous power of photosynthesis. Such is the importance of Phytonutrients – the Green Power.

Now, as far as we know, all *edible* plants contain nutrients, and Phytonutrient is the collective name for these. But not all of them are equal – some, like sweet potatoes, contain more carbohydrates than others, a few are very hot like chilli and curry, and others are very acidic like lemons and lime, and then there are very bitter ones like Chinese bitter melon. But all of them not only contribute nutrients to your body with special benefits which you can't obtain from animal meats, but they also make for a tasty meal if you know how to cook them with spices and condiments.

One of the cookbooks that has impressed me most, is *Land of Fish and Rice,* written by Fuchsia Dunlop, a trained chef who studied in China in the mid-1990s. She is exceptionally appreciative of the refined yet delicately subtle cuisine popular in regions south of the Yangze River; and in her book, which is full of pictures of the cuisine, only twenty pages are devoted to meat and poultry, while vegetable dishes taken up over two hundred pages. The books shows absolutely convincingly that vegetable cuisine can be produced in a hundred different yet appealing ways, which are marvellously tasty and look great.

First of all, I am going to show you a list of them, categorised in alphabetical order so they can be found easier. And under some of the well-known ones you will find up-to-date information on their nature, texture, main chemicals, and the best way to prepare them to make a tasty cuisine.

We will try to make the list as comprehensive as possible, with useful information from current books and works by reputable nutritionists and food scientists, with particular attention on the important and commonly available varieties available on the market.

Green Leafy Vegetables

Caution: all vegetables, melons, beans and peas required some cleaning and washing under the kitchen tap, or in a sink to be more thorough, to wash away sands, soil and various unwanted substance from the farm even though they look fresh and clean.

Before you purchase green vegies, try to feel and handle to make sure they feel firm, crispy and not limp or soft. Inspect the cut ends of the stems which should be uniformly fresh, green, not dry nor showing whitened fibrous changes. All the stems should snap with crispy sound.

And always try to get to the market in the early morning when it is just open. As farm suppliers usually harvest the vegies before dawn and truck the produce to the market shops before they are open. So if you are the early bird, you get the good 'worm' – the freshest vegies.

All the green parts of vegetables are heavily endowed with Chlorophyll which is superimposed on the other colourful pigments called Carotenoids. There are over at least 600 types of them isolated from fruits and vegies, all fat soluble and structurally related to Vitamin A (we'll look into this in more detail later). Chlorophyll is the green pigment of porphyrin/magnesium complex which enables green plants to absorb the energy from sunlight in order to synthesise sugar and carbon dioxide: a process known as photosynthesis. Among their other benefits, this substance seems to inhibit the chemicals in the cigarettes from causing cancer. It also as protects DNA from radiation damage.

Important vegetables and their properties

Baby bok choy

This is one of the most popular greens enjoyed by most Chinese, and quite familiar to many local Australians as well because they are now often commonly found on the restaurant menu or in the take-away box. If cooked well – best added to stir-fried garlic and ginger – the white juicy stem will remain crispy while the green leafy part becomes soft, tender with healthy taste of whatever sauce and good oil you put in. This green goes extremely well with most kinds of sliced meat and seafoods like prawns and scallop. Apart from the polyphenol, the green leaves are composed of a rich supply of chlorophyll.

This vegetable has a big brother the larger bok choy which is much bigger, coarser, perhaps more suitable for chop-suey dishes and soup.

Broccoli

This is one of the very popular vegies and belongs to the large Cruciferous group which includes cabbage, Brussels sprouts, cauliflower and kale. All of them have thiocyanates (sulphur containing chemicals/cells) which can protect us from GI tract cancers. They also help your liver to detox by stimulating more stage II detoxification enzymes. Broccoli contains Sulforaphane, some carotenoids (important plant chemicals rich in bright-coloured plants, carrots being the most obvious example), some Indoles and glutathione (a powerful anti-oxidant beneficial for liver, which helps it to detox the many harmful toxins and poisons which may wind up in your system). They are all some of the important chemicals, compounds and carotenoids as mentioned before.

Broccoli has a special chemical called Nicotinamide riboside (NR) a vital precursor of vit B 3 which your body will turn into

NAD. If you recall that David Sinclair has done a lot of research to try to discover more STACs to activate our longevity genes, and NAD (a form of Vit B3) is an outstanding STAC that is capable of boosting all the seven sirtuins in your body, as well as taking part in over five hundred different enzymes reactions. Normally your body can make the precursor NR from food like avocado, broccoli and cabbage. But the ability to do that would appear weaken as we get older and we may need NR as supplement (it is not cheap, about $80 per month on reliable brands).

In a 1996 Dutch studies from ninety-four clinical trials showed that broccoli, cabbage and cauliflower are the top vegies. Sixty-seven per cent of the studies, suggested that they had the most powerful protective effects against lung, stomach, colon and rectal cancers.

Although the cruciferous vegies taste rather 'pungent', they can still turn out quite pleasant. But you must stir-fry garlic/ginger first and add a pinch of sugar, soy sauce or oyster sauce. As long as you use good oil, at moderate temperature, and add some cooking wine and chicken stock, it makes a healthy tasty meal full of polyphenols which will protect your GI tract.

If you know what to use, home cooking is always healthy because you can control exactly what ingredients you have put in, like good quality oil.

Chinese Cabbage

This is the equivalent of the rounded cabbage you get from the supermarket, but there are some difference: it is somewhat longer, has a softer feel, is easier to cook, and cooks faster. It's best cooked with dried shrimps, sliced pork, and rice vermicelli, as a dish or in stock to make a flavoursome nutritious vegetable soup.

Choi sum

This Chinese plant is green from top to bottom and a favourite vegetable with Chinese families. It is usually tender if purchased in the right season, and although a bit more expensive, worth the extra cost. Outside the season, the stem tends to be tougher and more fibrous except for the tips which have yellow flowers.

All these greens, in addition to polyphenol, are rich in isoflavones (colourful pigments overshadowed by the intense green chlorophyll). These are very helpful to your cells and immune system.

Just the other day, I spotted a tray of nice green choi sum in a Chinese green grocery/supermarket. They were labelled correctly as 'Hong Kong choi sum' in small bunches. I can tell you this is the best quality choi sum, like I used to eat at home years ago before I came to Sydney and I can never forget how sweet and tender they are. So I bought a bunch home, cleaned them and put them into a large saucepan with some boiling chicken stock. In only a few minutes, the green is ready – so tender, fresh and sweet, without any spice. It brought back all my childhood memories of having this delicious green cooked at home.

Gui Lan

This is another really green vegie, similar to choi sum but with a thicker more meaty stem. It can be stir-fried or just cooked in a saucepan with stock. You can have it tender or crispy or in-between, depending on your individual preference. It also costs a bit more and tastes stronger than other greens, so you usually need a bit more sugar and cooking wine to bring out its healthy vegetable favour.

Lettuce – one of the most popular vegetable for salads and as a wrap with multiple tasty ingredients (as seen in 'San Choi Bao' in a Chinese banquet). It is a simple, attractive, easy to grow vegie found in backyard home gardens all over Australia. It just needs adequate watering and sunlight. No need for insecticide nor fertilisers. Lettuce is most suitable for all sorts of salad dishes for its crispiness and water content – usually a 'must' in summer cuisine.

Rocket

This is Mediterranean cruciferous plant, with the flowers and nowadays the leaves as salad. In terms of nutrition it certainly contains a lot more polyphenol than just lettuce alone. Best served raw with just a bit of extra virgin cold-pressed olive oil poured over it, with a pinch of pepper and salt or other spices, sprinkled on to taste. You can find them in a bunch or in a leaf mix in the chilled section of supermarkets. With a bit of care, they could be stored in your fridge, and last over a week. Please note : ideally most leafy greens should be cooked and eaten the same day after you have brought them from the market even though they can be kept fresh for a few days with plastic wrapping and stored in the vegetable compartment in the fridge.

Roots/Stems/bulbs or tubers

Some plants provide a lot of energy in the form of sugar and carbs. They perform this miracle by utilising sunlight and water, and hoard the chemical result in their bulbous roots with the intention of consuming them in adverse situations like drought. The common ones are carrots, potatoes, yams, beetroots, parsnips, radishes, sweet potatoes, turnips, celery, rhubarb, leeks, onions, bamboo, water-chestnuts, and asparagus. We are going to look at some of the ones with special features.

Asparagus

The young shoots are used as a spring vegetable, and there is another variety known as white asparagus. With their distinct favour, both are favourite greens in Europe. Chemical analysis shows that they are partly composed of several sulphur-containing chemicals. Asparagus has long enjoyed use in medicine for its diuretic property, and for its purported function as an aphrodisiac.

Asparagus is a good source of many vitamins – B6, C, E, K, thiamine, riboflavin, rutin, niacin, folic acid, and many minerals chiefly calcium magnesium, zinc, iron, phosphorus, potassium, copper, manganese and selenium. I also contains chromium, a trace mineral that regulates the ability of insulin to bring glucose from the blood into cells. It is pretty rich in the amino acid asparagine (which clearly gets its name from asparagus). One odd thing about this vegetable is that between forty and seventy per cent of eaters notice that their urine takes on a peculiar smell, which is thought to be due to the high sulphur content.

Bamboo
The young shoots can be used in dishes to give you sharp, crispy vegies in dishes such as chop-sue, which provides plenty of fibre.

Beetroot
This veggie is cultivated for its sugar content in colder climates where sugar cane is not suitable. Beetroot has been found to contain inorganic nitrate which can dilate blood vessels and lower blood pressure by up to 10mmHg for quite a few hours. Also found to reduce oxygen use during exercise, and beet and its juice are often used for better performance. Over-eating beets can cause kidney stones due to their high oxalate content.

Carrots
This is one of the many vegies containing beta carotene pigments which act as effective anti-cancer plant nutrients. There are at least over six hundred different carotenoids that have been discovered and there are doubtless many which are still unknown to science. In the vast plant kingdom of the earth there is a huge amount that is still undiscovered and which may never be fully catalogued. For example, my father spent his whole life studying medicinal plants and listed more than twenty-four thousand species just within Hong Kong's thirty square miles!

As well as being found in carrots, carotinoids are present in sweet potatoes, pumpkin, spinach, oranges, grapes, lemons, corn, apples, peaches, broccoli, tomatoes and many more plants. B-carotene, the most common form of carotene found in plants, is a powerful anti-oxidant, which can stimulate the immune system and T-cells.

Leeks and onions

These both belong to the same family. One study done in Shandong, China, found that those who ate more onions had forty per cent less gastric cancer. It has been discovered by Food Research International that red onions are most effective at killing human cancer cells due to their high levels of the antioxidants quercetin and antocyanin. Otherwise, with their appetising flavour, both are delicious stir-fried with eggs, sliced meats or just other crispy vegies.

Potatoes, Yam and sweet potatoes

All of these provide plenty of carbs for heat and energy, and each has its own distinct, pleasantly characteristic flavour. Potatoes are a staple in European diets. Sweet potatoes exist in at least three varieties – those with yellow flesh, red flesh and a purplish one. They are known to contain an array of vitamins and minerals including iron, calcium and selenium... The Okinawans lived for a long time on sweet potatoes during WWII when food shortages were severe due to fighting between Japanese and American soldiers. Fortunately, a villager returning from China had brought back sweet potatoes and propagated them widely as they discovered that the island's climate and soil conditions are ideal for this crop. Later the islanders erected a life-size statue of that villager in memory of his rescue effort.

According to the Wilcox brothers who have made numerous trips to Okinawa to study the locals' lifestyle, the islanders are particularly fond of eating the purple flesh variety which has been suspected to contain special phyto-nutrients which contribute to the islanders longer and healthier lifespan. From my survey of vegie markets in Sydney, all the above varieties of sweet potatoes are freely available. Even though the purple variety is moderately more expensive, when cooked it is more substantial and filling.

Parsnip, turnip, radish
All cooked and served as vegies like root/tuber food.

Capsicum
Crispy, meaty and vibrant these vegetables come in a variety of colours. They are native to the Americas, where they have been cultivated for thousands of years and are used in many cuisines. They are a good source of fibre and an excellent source of folate and vitamins A, E, B6 and C (the red capsicum naturally contains more of this than the other varieties).

Tomatoes
These are well known to be the major dietary source of lycopene which has been found to lower the risk of cancers of prostate, breast, GI tracts etc. They are also a great source of vitamin C, potassium, folate and vitamin K. Tomatoes are very easy to grow, can ripen to be very sweet and eaten like a fruit. To get the most benefit from tomatoes, it is best to cook them with good oil as the lycopene is not water soluble and locked inside the cell wall until it is cooked. You can also find a good source of lycopene from commercial tomatoes products like tomato juice, tomato sauce, or even Ketchup.

Tips for the home garden
If you want to you can grow your own vegetables. All you need is a small plot of good soil, well dug up and loose. It is best if mixed with compost. Plant the young vegies in, not too close to each other. Best to plant in spring in warmer states such as NSW and QLD, while in Victoria you need to wait till late spring when the temperature will warm up more.

Always water daily for about a week for the young vegies to settle and established, and then can be less frequent, depending on the rainfall over your region. Generally speaking, green leafy plants need more frequent watering to develop into juicy and succulent vegies, less for the hardy ones like peas and sweet potatoes.

Often one can plant shallots, spring onions, coriander and other spicess in between rows of your regular vegies, so that you can harvest them straight from your garden whenever you need them for stir fry or seafood etc. I must admit that I have missed my large garden plot in the back yard in Melbourne. I planted not only all different types of Chinese and local vegies including sugar pea, zucchini and pumpkin, I also put in many fruit trees such as golden delicious apples, apricot, cumquats, and a large, very productive edible fig which turned out hundreds of very sweet juicy fruits. These were incredibly attractive to the yellow-beaked birds and needed yearly protection with a huge net. It was good fun and awarding to share the harvested vegies and fruits with my family as well as our close friends.

Melons, sprouts, fungi and more

But natures goodies contain more than just veggies. These also have numerous benefits as well as adding some additional tasty treats to your table.

Alfalfa, bean sprouts

– Aussie alfalfa sprouts are a favourite add-on for dinner table salad. It has been shown to help lower cholesterol, and may have some benefits for blood-sugar control. It has got a high content of antioxidants, vitamin C and K, copper, folate and magnesium. Sprouting gives you up to 100 times more beneficial enzymes than are found in raw vegies because the rapidly growing sprouts need them. They have also plenty of enzyme inducers to protect against chemical carcinogens. Sprouting increases the vitamin and mineral content of nuts and seeds, particularly vitamin B and C, and carotene. The process helps break down anti-nutrients, enzyme inhibitors and makes the digestion and absorption by our guts much easier and more comfortable.

The main Chinese sprouts are from soybeans and green beans and they are usually stir-fried with meat and with spring onions to enhance the flavour, the texture and the fibre content.

Bitter melon, Ghit-melon, Si-melon, and Winter melon
These are the four most common Chinese melons. The first three are usually for stir-fry, and the last one to make soup.

The bitter melon has been found to lower blood sugar due to a chemical acting like insulin, which helps bring glucose into the cells for production of energy and move glucose to your liver, muscles for use.

The melon has to be prepared by cutting it open, scooping out the seeds and pith with a small spoon and cutting it into slices. It is then parboiled for a few minutes to rid it of its bitterness, then stir fried with the usual ingredients and spices like garlic, spring onions, lean pork slices and soy sauces or whatever you fancy.

The winter melon is a big rounded like a watermelon. It may serve as a mild diuretic when ingested in soup.

Mushrooms and fungi
These fabulous products of nature have been an extremely popular source of food in Asian countries for thousands of years, and have also played an important role in medicine. The Asian attitude to food is similar to that expressed by Hippocrates, the ancient Greek physician who said that 'food be your medicine and medicine be your food'.

Fungi, black and white
The black fungus, also popularly known as 'cloud ear' fungus by the Chinese, are not generally consumed by Europeans but they have been a common and important ingredient in Chinese cuisine and medicine for centuries. It looks and feels like dried up crumpled leaves until soaked in water overnight which leads it to expand into a large soft, crispy and chewy vegetable. It tastes almost neutral before being lightly stir-fried with sauces to bring out its full flavour and peculiar texture. It is found to have

extremely high iron content, very beneficial to people with anaemia. It is also rich in protein, vitamins and polysaccharides which help prevent inflammation particularly in mucous tissue and inhibits a key enzyme responsible for Alzheimer's disease. It can also lower blood cholesterol, triglycerides, and inhibit platelet clumping or thrombosis. The rich B2 is a strong anti-oxidant to protect the cells as well. On the whole, it seems to have many beneficial effects for our health.

It goes well with many dishes, mainly to add some unusual shiny black vegie and the unforgettable texture. There are a few other varieties like white fungus and snow fungus which can be transformed into a favourite Chinese dessert (mainly prepared at home, occasionally served in good restaurants).

Mushrooms have many varieties, the common ones available on the market are large field mushrooms, small, cultured button mushrooms, shiitake, reishi, maitake, oyster mushrooms and king mushrooms from Korea. There are estimated to be up to over two hundred and seventy varieties eaten in China. They are all tasty, soft but chewy, with an excellent refined flavour if prepared well, and are often used as a main ingredient in expensive dishes of prawns and scallops.

The type called maitake mushroom has recently been discovered by Japanese scientists to be able to directly activate various immune cells (killer cells, macrophages, killer T-cells etc.) to attack cancer and even the Aids virus as well.

An extract named PSK derived from other mushrooms, has been approved for consumers by the Japanese FDA and sold widely all over Japan and Europe.

Shiitake is another outstanding mushroom – it has two times as much fibre and protein as others sold in supermarkets, and it is also found to contain plenty of calcium, and vitamins D and B. It can help lower blood pressure and cholesterols.

So mushroom lovers not only enjoy their favourite delicacy gastronomically, but they also are enjoying a great many health benefits.

Algae, Seaweed

These gifts from the oceans and seas are found to have sixty per cent of protein by weight, enough to supply all eight types of our body's need of essential amino acids and gamma linolenic acid, one of the good oils. They are also rich in chlorophyll, B6 and B12, and contain a great deal of carotenoid in concentrated form, near ten times more than carrots and they have been found to prevent some pre-malignant skin condition like leukoplakia on the lips and mucus membrane.

Chlorella

A fresh-water algae, rich in chlorophyll, vitamins and minerals.

Kelp

This is a brown seaweed, said to help bring down your BP and lipids, so it should be healthy food for your CVS. Also found by Japanese researchers to be able to reduce the risk of cancer of the colon. Kelp, like jellyfish, is usually sold in slender slices kept in clean water in sealed bags, obtainable in some health food shops or in Chinese grocery shop. Kelp has no taste, it's just crispy and chewy like jellyfish, and can go into any cuisine cooked with a good sauce.

Nuts, Seeds and Legumes

The main characteristics common to all of these is that they are rich in protein, carbs, fibre and oils (mainly Omega 6 oil). They are useful also as a hunger stopper – it is recommended that you have just a handful of them anytime if you are on a diet and conscious of your weight as their caloric value is so low as to present no threat to your regime.

Some of them need to be mentioned for special features and nutritional values as follows:

Almonds

These originated in Iran, but now the US is the biggest grower. Almonds help with weight loss, lower LDL and ameliorate arthritis. They are rich in vitamin E, magnesium and potassium. They are a nutritious nut that make a great snack.

Brazil nuts

Unsurprisingly, these come from a South American tree, which is one of the largest and longest-lived trees in the Amazon rainforest. The fruit and its nutshell is large, up to two kilograms in total weight. They have a diverse content of micronutrients, in particular a high amount of Selenium which is a potent anti-oxidant and immunostimulant that helps reduce the risk of GI tract cancer by sixty-three per cent and prostate cancer by seventy per cent according to a 1996 study in the Journal of the American Medical Association. They also protect against mercury poisoning from seafood – which could happen if you feed on large fish like tuna and swordfish etc. And if you do, it is advisable to see your GP to have your blood mercury level checked and change your choice of fish to smaller fish varieties like sardines, bream, barramundi, etc.

Pumpkin Seeds

These are packed full of anti-oxidants, healthy fats (six of which are Omega 6), magnesium and zinc. So they can improve your heart and prostate health. Twenty-eight grams (one ounce) contains: Fibres 1.7 gm, carbs 5 gm, protein 7 gm, fat 13 gm, vit K 18% of the RDI, iron 23% of the RDI, 14% of the RDI of zinc, as well as much manganese 42% and magnesium 37%.

Sesame Seeds

These may be the base for the oldest condiment known to man. They are highly valued for their oil which is exceptionally resistant to rancidity. They are an excellent source of copper, and a very good source of manganese as well as calcium, iron, zinc, and selenium. The rich copper gives relief for rheumatoid arthritis, while the others support vascular and respiratory health, bone health, and the calcium helps prevent colon cancer and osteoporosis.

Sesame seeds, whether eaten whole or in the pulverised powder form, including the black variety, and tahini (the hulled and unhulled paste) are all available from supermarkets and Asian grocery shops. I have found them easily mixed in milk with whatever breakfast cereals, and of course as ingredient and condiment to add subtle flavour and texture to the cuisine,

Soybeans
This is the only legume with outstanding phytonutrients. It has been cultivated in China for over five thousand years and was later adopted by other Asian nations. Its popularity has spread all over the world and particularly to the US which has been exporting tonnes and tonnes of it to China. Soybeans can be cooked and eaten like any other beans such as chickpeas and green beans. The Chinese are particularly fond of turning it into curdled form (tofu) for easy stir-frying, or tofu skin or concentrated dry tofu, all different forms to facilitate cooking and consumption

Soybeans can also be turned into a dairy milk substitute. They are available either in re-constituted form in the supermarket with a healthy proportion of proteins and fats (mostly PUFA or polyunsaturated fatty acids). They are rich in vitamins, particularly vitamin D and calcium: up to 400 mg per serve, even more than dairy milk. It can be bought as freshly produced soy-milk in two-litre plastic bottles sold in Chinese grocery stores – a refreshingly nutritious drinks in its undiluted form.

Soybeans are composed of thirty per cent carbs, thirty-eight per cent protein and eighteen per cent oil – most of it being unsaturated good oil. They are a rich source of various vitamins, minerals and beneficial plant compounds such as isoflavones and phytoestrogens which are very weak oestrogens (about one thousandth as strong as human oestrogen). So, in a normal human, these weak oestrogens will stick to the oestrogen receptors of human cells in the breast and ovary, as well as prostate and colon, thus blocking the chance for oestrogen related cancer cells to stick onto those organs and be nourished and grown.

Yet, at all times, the soybean phytoestrogens are too weak to cause any significant symptoms in the host such as hot flushes, migraines, weight increase, etc. that often are present in hormone irregularities.

Soybeans, among all other legumes, are the only ones found to contain all the nine essential amino acids our body requires so that you don't need to force yourself to eat meat to get them, which is a great benefit to the pure vegetarians. Because of those many special features and contents, soybeans have been studied intensely in recent years to further explore their benefit for our heart health.

Results from a meta-analysis of thirty-eight clinical studies, published in the prestigious medical journal the *New England Journal of Medicine* in 1995, concluded that consuming more soy-proteins resulted in significantly lowered cholesterol and LDL when compared to subjects who consumed animal proteins. The studies were later followed up by the American FDA and the UK health authority, who both strongly supported the findings.

In a European study, Genistein, being one of the three isoflavones/phytoestrogens from soybeans, was found to be a potent anti-cancer chemical which displayed two very important influences. Firstly, as cancer cells cannot grow without nutrition from the host cells, they try to take advantage of our body's natural ability to grow new blood vessels, a process which is called angiogenesis. It is mainly designed for the purpose of repairing damaged tissue after operations or injuries so they can live on and grow – how clever! But this Genistein has been found to be a powerful blocker of angiogenesis in lab cultures. Under normal conditions, the normal type of angiogenesis will be initiated after injuries, surgery, etc, because the feed-back mechanism of the body can sense and distinguish between the normal angiogenesis from the haphazard type initiated by cancer cells. And you need genistein therapy in cancer cases.

Secondly cancer cells often try to fool our immune cells by producing some 'stress protein' to confuse the immune cells in the hope that they cannot be recognised. But Genistein also suppress such proteins being produced. As you can see, Genistein from soybeans cuts off the cancer cells from their angiogenesis and prevents them from being camouflaged against the killer cells from the immune system. So the budding cancer will clearly be destroyed well before it grows too big. This cancer eliminating ability of Genistein has been confirmed at the Johns Hopkins University lab in 1998. In 1996, researchers found Genistein could block a particular enzyme – Tyrosin kinase – to stop prostate cancer-cell growth.

Looking at all the wonderful plant nutrients and isoflavones provided by them it is clear that the soybean is something of a miracle food. And yet it is among the most affordable and widely available foods we have at our service. If anything is recommended to fulfill the hypocritic exhortation that 'food be your medicine, and medicine be your food' it is this humble legume.

Fruits

In general, all fruits are sweet and colourful, which indicates that they are full of B-carotenoids. They are rich in carbs and vitamin C, and all or most of the fat-soluble vitamins A, E, D, K, minerals and most of the phyto-nutrients like polyphenols. Vitamin A in high concentration is very protective for your vision and skin, while vitamin C is a strong anti-oxidant capable of blocking nitrites from becoming nitrosamine (a carcinogen). They also lower the risk of cancer of the oesophagus and stomach.

Let's look at some of the fruits with special features and explore deeper into their health benefits.

Avocado

This large dark green fruit of several varieties is actually dubbed the "buttery fruit" by the Chinese because its pale-yellow soft meat is oily and can be readily spread on bread or toast like butter, with the benefit of it being cholesterol free. It contains plenty of good oils formed of monounsaturated fatty acids, and twenty vitamins and minerals. Together with the cruciferous vegies like broccoli and cabbage, avocado contains NR, the important precursor of B3, for the body to turn it into NAD as a vital chemical (one of the STACs to activate our longevity genes).

It can be eaten raw, as a breakfast appetiser, using a spoon to scoop up the soft meat, perhaps after light sprinkling it with pepper and salt to enhance its subtle flavour. Any remaining portion has to be covered up or wrapped up with a freezer bag to prevent contact of air as the meat can become oxidized and take on a yellowish brown colour fairly quickly. It helps to improve your digestion, and reduce depression, protect your CVS, reduce body weight, control NIDDM, and it gives some protection against cancer too!

Apricot

This soft sweet fruit is surprisingly very healthy. It is packed full not only with vitamins A, C and E, but also contains plenty of polyphenols and anti-oxidants, notably important ones like lutein, zeaxanthin, b-carotene, catechin and quercetin – the latter two are anti-oxidants well-known for protecting the retinas of your eyes and helping to maintain normal vision. All those flavonoids (plant nutrients/chemicals) will help regulate NIDDM and CVD, also capable of reducing about fifty per cent of inflammation whatever the cause – so it can play an important role in combating diseases that produce inflammation like arthritis, myositis, over-use soft tissue inflammation etc. So it is also protective for the skin against UV damage. Apricot, among its other virtues, stands apart from other fruits in that it contains both soluble and insoluble fibres, but is high in soluble fibres which dissolve in the gut to form pectin, gums, and long chains of sugar called polysaccharides which will improve your gut function by serving as ideal nourishment to the friendly bacteria so they work better and lower the absorption of sugar and cholesterol. It has been analysed that one cup of sliced apricots will provide up to ten per cent of the recommended daily intake of vitamins and fibres.

Kiwi fruit

Also known as "Chinese gooseberry" the special feature of this fruit is that it has an abundant amount of vitamin C, in addition to vitamin K, E, folate, fibres and anti-oxidants. It is also said to be a 'sleep inducer', which might be worth a try for people troubled by insomnia, as part of their practise of good sleep hygiene.

Mandarin-orange

This fruit, native to China and SE Asia, now is cultivated worldwide, in quite a few varieties including hybrids. In 2017, the world produced over thirty-three million tonnes of mandarin-oranges, with China leading production with fifty-four per cent of the total. The fruit is soft and tastes sweet with a tinge of tanginess, contain thirteen per cent carbs and thirty-two per cent vitamin C. But the Chinese keep the peel for special purposes – using the fresh peel in cooking and baking for its essential oil, and the dried peel as medicine to regulate the 'Chi' and to help to improve digestion.

Because of the pun (same pronunciation as 'gold' in Chinese) and the golden yellow colour to match, the fruit has for centuries been held up as symbolising good fortune and good luck by Chinese, Japanese and most Asians all over the world. This lends it an appealing cultural significance which is enjoyed along with its benefits as a food and medicine!

Mango

This fruit is often dubbed 'King of Fruits' because the fruit is incredibly sweet and juicy, with an appetising aroma. Just one bite of the succulent meat and you will be a mango lover forever! This fruit tree has been cultivated for over four thousand years in South East Asia and has over hundreds of varieties with their own individual shape, taste and colour. It is no surprise too that the mango is called the king of fruits because it is packed with nutrients, minerals, vitamins and powerful anti-oxidants.

One cup of mango meat has just under one and a half grams of protein, twenty-five grams of carbs and six grams of fibre. It is very rich in vitamin C: up to sixty-seven per cent of the recommended daily intake. It also contains the RDI of the following: twenty per cent of copper; eighteen per cent of folate; twelve percent of vitamin B6, ten per cent of vitamins A and E; and six and a half per cent of vitamin B5, niacin, vitamin K, potassium, riboflavin, manganese, thiamine and magnesium, It even contains small amounts of calcium, iron and selenium. Mango is richly supplied with anti-oxidants and contains over twelve kinds, including the familiar lutein and zeaxanthin which help protect eyesight, and a supremely powerful anti-oxidant called mangiferin which is only found in mangos. In addition, it contains several types of amylase – a digestive enzyme. So, armed with all these vitamins, minerals, enzymes and powerful anti-oxidants, those who eat a lot of mangos are expected to have enhanced immune systems, better digestive and heart health, better protected eyesight, and a lower risk of cancers of the colon, lungs, prostate and breast. What a wonderful gift from the plant kingdom! So yummy to eat, yet loaded with so many health benefits. Put mango on your required eating list, and consume at least a few every week while the they are in season and comparatively cheap.

Paw Paw

Also known as "papaya" the tree that bears this fruit was originally cultivated in central America and is nowadays spreading all over the globe. It has large fruit, which are best eaten when they ripen to yellow/orange, or you can consume an excellent variety with red meat, from Queensland and Thailand. In one small 150 grams of fruit, you can find 15 grams of carbs, 3 gm of fibre and 1gm of protein, and they are loaded with vitamin C, antioxidants and carotenoids, especially Lycopene.

Somehow the antioxidants and lycopene in paw paw are better absorbed by your body than the same chemicals contained in other fruits and vegetables – quite likely due to the powerful digestive enzymes called chymopapain and papain which help the gut to digest tough meat fibres. In some parts of the world, pawpaw is often used to treat constipation and irritable bowel syndrome with success. The rich supply of vitamin C and lycopene support heart health, suppress inflammation, which is easily checked by testing the level of CRP.

Japan, is a country whose population has prevalent gastric problems, and its scientists have done a great deal of research into pawpaw enzymes and produced numerous patented medications for the public. Many of them appear to work well and compare favourably with some more expensive products imported from the US.

Pineapple

Like most others cited beforehand, this strange-looking fruit which originates in Latin America is packed full of nutrients, vitamins and antioxidants, all rated +++. For example a serving of two hundred grams they can provide a high per cent of the recommended daily intake of both vitamin C and manganese.

The whole fruit is actually made up of multiples of small fruit, each one being marked with an 'eye' on the hard skin that needs to be scooped out or dug out. The pineapple has been discovered to contain a special enzyme – Bromelain – a complex extract from the stem and the core, found to have a wide variety of health benefits. It is anti-inflammatory, helps the digestive system, is protective of the immune system, slows down coagulation, and suppresses the growth of certain tumours.

Berries and grapes

There are over four hundred types of berries in various colours but black and purple predominate. They share the characteristic virtue of being packed full of antioxidants, vitamins, minerals, and many plant nutrients. Blueberries appears to be the champion, as recommended by the FDA, due to their high level of antioxidants.

Grape varieties are even more numerous – over several thousands of them, according to Tom Stevenson's book on wine throughout the world, partly due to the cultivation of grafted varieties, the cross-fertilised ones, hybrids, clones etc.

In general, one hundred grams of grapes contain a hundred and ninety milligrams of potassium; sixteen grams of sugar; six per cent recommended daily intake of vitamin C; five per cent RDI of vitamin B6; one per cent RDI of calcium.

Eating grapes gives you the following benefits, according to the Cleveland Clinic:

- Helps your immune system due to the high content of vitamin C as a strong antioxidant.

- Protects against heart disease due to resveratrol which is a well-known polyphenol that reduces inflammation and LDL the bad cholesterol.
- Helps to push back the ageing process due to the content of resveratrol and many other polyphenols such as catechins, quercetin and anthocyannins. Together they stimulate Sirtuin (SirT1, the longevity gene) and block the growth of cancer cells to give us a longer and healthier lifespan.
- Other minor benefits are maintaining bone health with their calcium content and high potassium (K), and their ability to lower blood sugar by enhancing insulin sensitivity.

Herbs and spices

Every day or two most of us need to go shopping to bring back food for our family. Apart from breakfast cereals, breads and milk, we need to shop for vegetables more frequently for their freshness and nutrition. When vegies are stored in the fridge for more than a few days, particularly the green leafy types, they might get dehydrated or go yellow, meaning they are losing the green chlorophyll and some other plant nutrients. That could be one of the reasons many busy working couples are discouraged from eating vegies. However, you just need to adjust your routine in some ways so that you can do some snap shopping during your lunch time, or after work as most reputable supermarkets operate till late for the convenience of working people.

At the beginning of this chapter, we listed most of the commonly consumed plants available on the market, like lovely lettuce, baby bok choy, nutritious cruciferous broccoli, cauliflower, spinach, exceptionally healthy root vegies like carrots, onions and sweet potato, and a long list of important locally grown fruits, with Australian grown grapes being given prominent mention for their internationally recognised excellent quality.

All that having been said, we must now introduce those great culinary helpers – the spices, herbs and condiments. They are all sourced from plants that have been consumed in part or whole for thousands of years, often not just as cooking ingredients but also as therapeutic medicines – such are the wonderful gifts to humans from the plant kingdom.

At the beginning of this book, I have taken my readers through the five world-famous blue zones of Bapan in China, Okinawa in Japan, Sardinia in Italy, Loma Linda in California and Costa Ricca in mid-America. We know their all very different lifestyles, we have found out the bulk of what they eat most, but we are quite ignorant of the wonderful herbs and spices in their cuisines – and that is basically very important, because many of the spices and culinary herbs exert powerful therapeutic effects on health and the immune system. One may wonder if regular ingestion of some herbs and spice possibly contributes to their energy and good health and helps add a few more years to their lifespan.

So I have made an effort to check up their culinary habits from the most updated work and studies, and have found that the followings are the most commonly chosen herbs and spices, which are used in almost every dish consumed at lunch and dinner. I will list them all, and will pick some of the most important ones for extended examination.

Commonly used herbs and spices in centenarian diets as follows:

- basil
- parsley
- thyme
- oregano
- bay leaves
- garlic
- mint
- rosemary
- saffron (only commonly used in Sardinia)

- cumin
- turmeric
- coriander
- cardamom
- chilli
- soy
- miso
- vanilla
- Chinese 5-spice
- ginger
- sage
- salt and pepper

Now, for more detailed descriptions on essential ones.

Basil

This herb belongs in the same family as the peppermint plant. It is hailed as the king of herbs, and has been used worldwide in cuisines, originated in the tropics. The health benefits come from its flavonoids and volatile oils, and it is now studied all over the world for its unique properties. One of Basil's volatile oils is called eugenol, known for its anti-inflammatory effects, which make it protective of the body. Basil extract has proven effective in fighting breast cancer with its programmed cell death, and its high level of lutein can also reduce the risk of the disease. Basil's antioxidant is also believed by many scientists to help reduce damage on inner linings of coronary arteries from free radicals due to the phytochemicals in its essential oils.

Basil extract, especially that derived from a variety called 'holy basil', is found to be effective in controlling blood-sugar levels, although exactly what compound in the extract is exerting this effect is still being researched. Basil has quite a few volatile essential oils to protect itself from bacterial infection, each species of basil has different concentrations of eugenol, citral, etc. Lemon basil, for example, has more limonene and citral phytochemicals. Basil has long been used in traditional medicine to fight bacteria. These oils have also been found to lower blood triglyceride and LDL.

In addition to all this, basil has been used, particularly in India, for combating arthritis and its pain, it is reportedly able to reduce pain by over seventy per cent and to improve digestion as it balances acid and is friendly to good gut bacteria.

Bay leaves – a very commonly used herbal leaf, usually only on leaf is used in any kind of dish, to give it a distinctive flavour and fragrance, but the leaf is usually removed before serving. They are a rich source of vitamins A and C, iron, potassium, calcium and magnesium. They have been proven to be beneficial in the treatment of migraines. They do have a known side effect, which is drowsiness, and should therefore not be taken with sedatives.

Cinnamon
Fund in Chinese five-spice, it is obtained from the inner bark of several tree species which come under the classification of Cinnamomum. It is used mainly as an aromatic condiment and flavouring additive in a wide variety of cuisines, including both sweet or savoury dishes. It is rich in dietary fibre, iron, calcium and potassium. It is the ingredients in Chinese 5-spice powder that gives the distinctive, appetising aroma of roast duck, chicken and BBQ pork.

Chinese 5-spice
This is the most versatile spice used by the Chinese in a wide variety of cuisines that give very pleasant, appetite arousing aroma, commonly in their roasted meats, BBQ meats, and stir-fried cuisines. It is also a good addition to soup and tea. As the name suggests, it is a combination of five familiar powdered spices: Chinese Cinnamon, Cloves, Fennel, Star anise, and Szechuan peppercorns.

Of the five spices, star anise is distinguished by its rich variety of flavonoids and polyphenolic compounds: it has at least six major ones, including the well-known Quercetin, that may contribute to the antioxidant, anti-inflammatory and anti-microbial properties of this spice. Some animal studies indicate that star anise may even possess anti-cancer properties such as suppressing tumour growth and reducing its size. Naturally more research is required to discover its potential in supporting human health.

Chilli

Chilli peppers originated from Mexico which is famous for the inexpensive dish called *chili con carne*, which is a sort of chilli spiced meat dish. The chemical content of chilli is capsaicin, which is used as an analgesic in topical ointment to relieve pain and even arthritic pain. Spicy foods like chilli peppers may keep your heart healthy, when we consider the lower levels of LDL found in people who eat red chilli peppers regularly, but more well-conducted studies are needed to evaluate this properly. Otherwise, Chilli has been one of the most used hot spices and most welcome condiments in SE Asia where people use it in almost every dish to enhance the flavour and help stimulate the appetite. Some species of chilli could be so hot that just a small piece would give you a feeling of swallowing a burning charcoal all the way down from your throat and these can make you very sick. So you need to be very alert about the type of hot food you are grazing on if you go on a culinary tour in the SE Asia.

Coriander

This cute, lovely herb, also called Chinese parsley, as it is related to parsley, carrots and celery, is used in almost all Asian cuisines for its distinctive aroma. Usually the whole plant is used, chopped, mixed with chopped spring onions or shallots, and sprinkled all over steamed seafood dishes like fish, scallops and prawns. But, in fact, due to its fresh taste and pleasing colour, this herb is frequently presented to gourmet eaters spread on Chinese dishes among the topping greens. It can also come in seeds and oils. Its main therapeutic effect is in lowering blood sugar, and, in fact, people on diabetic medication should practise caution with coriander as its effect is quite similar to one of the diabetic medications, glibenclamide (Daonil). It offers quite a few good antioxidants like quercetin, and tocopherols (vitamin E) which are good for fighting cancer and inflammation and boosting the immune system. Coriander extract and seeds appear to help to reduce salt intake and lower BP and LDL by acting like a diuretic. Studies on rats have shown that coriander leaves and extract improved memory which suggests that they could afford some protection against Alzheimer's and Parkinson's diseases due to its anti-inflammatory properties.

It also helps in IBS (irritable bowel syndrome – a very annoying condition of alternating tummy pain, diarrhoea and constipation) and GI digestion. Its extract is used as appetite stimulant in traditional Iranian medicine. It has antimicrobial compounds that can fight common gastroenteritis.

Turmeric
Also known as "curcumin", this spice belongs to the ginger family, and has been used as a spice for many centuries in both China and India. Indian Ayurvedic medical practitioners have long used it as a herbal medicine to treat GI disorders and skin cancers. As turmeric is the major component of curry (another popular spice), it comes as no surprise that India is the largest producer of turmeric.

Way back in my childhood years in Hong Kong, curry dishes were already among the most popular and sought after spicy foods, being held equally in favour as soy sauce, oyster sauce and BBQ pork. As kids we craved the distinctly appetising aroma and flavour of a good curry.

L Braun and Marc Cohen, of RMIT University, Melbourne have described in detail how, about forty years ago, an increasing number of studies on this spice shed a great deal of light on its nature and effects. Now curcumin has been discovered to be an extremely powerful anti-cancer agent. This was shown in a study of many cases regarding nasty oral cancers which were not responding to conventional treatments such as surgery, chemotherapy and radiation. In one study in India, involving sixty-two such cases, as described in Dr Gaynor's *Cancer Prevention Program*, only eighteen months of treatment with curcumin preparations, most of the nasty symptoms had been reduced by ninety per cent and the size of the cancers had been reduced by fifty per cent.

In some of the studies done on lab animals by Indian scientists recently, curcumin has displayed the power to inhibit the growth of cancers of the breast, stomach and colon. Clearly, many of the methods by which cancer can be initiated, progress and spread, seem to have been blocked by the variety of polyphenols in curcumin.

This spice has also been investigated and found to possess a powerful antioxidant and anti-inflammatory effect. As a strong antioxidant, it also acts by scavenging free radicals, modulate glutathione peroxidase (a strong oxidative chemical) and generally acting like vitamin E. Its potent anti-inflammatory action could be applied to ameliorate neurodegenerative diseases such as Alzheimer's, Parkinson's diseases, MS (multiple sclerosis), asthma, osteoarthritis, NIDDM, colitis, etc. Curcumin exerts its beneficial effects on metabolic syndrome by increasing insulin sensitivity, disrupting adipogenesis (fat production), bringing down HBP. It can also modulate expression of genes and enzymes in lipoprotein metabolism, reducing TGL and LDL, while pushing up HDL. This illustrates both how complex battling metabolic syndrome is and how many beneficial aspects there are to this wonder spice.

This is one important note which needs to be heeded: curcumin taken by itself does not give you much in the way of health benefits because of its poor bioavailability (L Braun & M

Cohen's *Herbs and Natural Supplements*) even though it can be taken in high doses of up to twelve thousand milligrams per day (as approved by the FDA). But if some other spices are added to it, the effects will be a huge surprise, for example, if black pepper to be mixed with it, the bioavailability will be increased by two thousand per cent! That may be the reason people just use curry powder (curcumin is the major ingredient in mixed spice powder) as the major culinary condiment in cooking – it is far easier and tastier too.

Ginseng

This is easily the most famous health supplement known in Asian countries, with its iconic label showing the picture of the herb which shows that it's shape is closely similar to that of the human form. Even the illiterate can pick the ginseng tea package without seeing the name. In most people's minds, ginseng is considered a general tonic for the body and believed to impart protection against colds and flu's, stimulate the immune system and increase your energy level.

But there are several types of ginseng. The true plant is called panax ginseng, often called Chinese ginseng, which is widely grown in China, Korea and Japan, which as the only variety used by the Chinese and Koreans for over five thousand years that has been thoroughly studied. There is also an American variety but not much is known about it. Korean scientists had recently done a study on several thousand people by using ginseng extract known to contain dozens of ginseng compounds (saponins) and found that those taking ginseng longer with larger doses had fifty per cent less chance of getting cancer, depending upon dose and duration. The type of cancers most responsive to the protective effects of ginseng were those of the upper GI tract, pancreas and oesophagus.

As a general tonic, the Chinese take ginseng to improve memory as it has a kind of plant-based stimulant to increase brain cell activity and concentration. So it could be useful for combatting Alzheimer's and to push back ageing. Ginseng has anti-

216

inflammatory effects and can help reduce headache and stress, provide menopausal relief, improve mood and act as an immune booster against colds and flus.

One word of caution: find out the most reputable distributer and purchase only after their reliability and the price have been checked. Avoid buying online until you are sure the brand and source are trustworthy. Or see if you can get recommendation from a friend or current users.

Ginger

This delightful cuisine ingredient, used world-wide, has recently been found by Japanese scientists to contain up to fourteen types of phenol, or more, which act as potent antioxidants. These chemicals, called gingerol and zingerone, are stronger than vitamin E, which is probably why ginger has long been used to preserve foodstuff from becoming spoiled due to oxidative stress.

Ginger is traditionally used by the Chinese in all stir-fry cooking and is a must for seafood cuisine as it turns any 'fishy' taste into peppery aromatic flavour. Ginger spiced cuisine is not only appetite arousing, it is also beneficial for ailments of the GI tract and has long been utilized as a herbal medicine for constipation, diarrhoea, and other disorders. In 2017, researchers at the University of Bologna found that ginger root demonstrated impressive beneficial effects on the smooth muscle of the intestine, and this is believed to be due to its gingerols.

Ginger has also been found by researchers in Cleveland to be able to reduce skin tumours on mice, which may indicate that the phenols inside ginger are potent anti-cancer phytochemicals though this possibility needs to be further researched. Shogoals, another chemical found in ginger (which is also called Shokyo by the Japanese), has been studied in 2015 and found to promote strong anti-cancer stem-cell activity and shows promise as a means of suppressing cancer-cell growth in pancreatic, ovarian and prostate cancers.

A 2013 study by the Zanjan Metabolic Disease Centre suggested that ginger helps reduce insulin resistance, reduce sugar in circulation, improve beta-cell function and lipid profiles, so adding ginger into food regularly for people with NIDDM should be a healthy supplement.

As ginger's phenols are powerful antioxidants as well as anti-inflammatory, it has been studied along these lines which suggest it has potential benefits for asthma, menopausal pain, rheumatoid arthritis, neurodegenerative disease and MS.

I am pretty sure more research is in the pipeline for this fascinating, wonderful universal spice. The breaking news on ginger is that recently the price has gone up over 100% (from $30 to up to $70 per kilo) due to covid-19 and a poor harvest. Still not that expensive in comparison to vanilla beans which cost $8 for only one bean.

Garlic

This extremely popular seasoning has been known and used for 5000 years both as culinary spice and as herbal medicine. It is extensively cultivated in China and Iran. In its bulb, the herbal medicinal effects come mainly from its sulphur compound which includes allicin and seems to exert a moderate effect in bringing down lipids. In a recently reported meta-analysis, it has been found to lower total cholesterol (++), LDL (+), TGL (++), and result in atherosclerotic plaque reduction (++) compared with placebo group.

Garlic has also proven moderate anti-platelet properties capable of prolonging bleeding time of your body and it is advisable to refrain from consuming garlic before a blood test. L Pasteur, the researcher who introduced 'Pasteurisation' to milk, found garlic to be an anti-microbial chemical, which led to a garlic preparation being used as an antiseptic to prevent gangrene in both WWI and WWII.

Recently in a Shandong study, in China, in 1987, it was found that those who ate a lot of garlic in their meals forty per cent less gastric cancer than average. In another review of literature by John Pinto of the Memorial S-K cancer centre, in 1997, altogether twenty studies, reported that garlic consumption may help prevent at least six types of cancer – breast, colon, stomach and oesophagus, prostate and skin.

Known as one of the most popular global spices, garlic is almost always used either on its own in Western cooking (or together with other condiment like coriander, bay leaves and rosemary) but, in Asian cuisines, the chef never fails to pair it with ginger and shallots, in any stir-fry, to bring out and enhance the full flavour of the food.

With its added benefit to heart health, there is no reason for you to forget crushing garlic cloves into your everyday cooking. Garlic is now very cheap as China is a fantastic grower and their garlic cloves are seen flooding the market by the bagful. But you also have the choice to search for the locally produced ones at somewhat more expensive cost but more fresh. Alternately, you can use the smaller, red-skin onion which may not taste so pungent as garlic.

Rosemary

This well-known plant, is a native in the Mediterranean region and traditionally used as a very common herb in many Western dishes, particularly with roasts, due to its special aromatic flavour. It is often paired with garlic, curcumin, cloves, organo, thyme, sage etc. The plant is hardy and easily grown.

Rosemary has also been used in many countries outside the Mediterranean region for centuries as a versatile medicinal herb due to its effects as an anti-bacterial, anti-NIDDM, anti-inflammatory, anti-diuretic, hepato-protective agent. Lately, it has been discovered to also act as an anti-cancer agent and have effects which are anti-thrombotic, meaning that it helps to prevent blood clotting.

In studies conducted in the 1990s, scientist discovered two powerful enzymes in rosemary, that inhibit tumours and the risky COX-2 from the prostaglandins. It has also been found to produce two other useful enzymes, glutathione and quinone, which are both formidable detoxifying enzymes.

Another research article in an Indian journal of complementary medicine, describes how a study into rosemary found that most of its pharmaceutical effects come from its special phenolic properties –and it appears to be a very promising therapeutic means to help combat Alzheimer's and Parkinson's diseases. Rosemary has also been approved by EU officials as safe and useful for food preservation due to its effective antioxidant nature.

Tea

This ubiquitous plant that has been providing the cheapest and healthiest daily drink for the general public for over five thousand years. Tea is made from the young leaves of the simple plant *Camellia sinensis* ('sinensis' meaning 'of Chinese origin'). China still remains the world's largest tea producer, ahead of Sri Lanka and India which also have extensive tea plantations in Assam and Darjeeling. Taiwan and Japan have followed suit recently.

Apart from China and the SE Asian nations, Britain and Western European countries have also been the biggest tea drinking population, importing and consuming almost one third of world's production. Particularly in England, and Australia too, a 'cuppa' or 'morning tea' is normally the short break being looked forward to by most workers, whether in the office, shops, schools, or on the farm. The short break provide workers the opportunity to relax and recover, as well as enjoy a chat. Tea has got some caffeine, enough to act as a mild stimulant, serving to help you feel rather refreshed after the 'cuppa'. And, astonishingly, tea supplies many other beneficial polyphenols to contribute to your good health and immune system.

Healthwise, tea is far better than coffee which has recently replaced much of the good habit of tea drinking. Coffee is more aromatic, but also far more addictive and more expensive. The coffee culture originated in the coffee houses in London and France in the old days, where it nurtured much high-spirited gossip and the discussion of literature and politics. These days, coffee culture has changed fundamentally to the Americanised commercial style, often run and controlled by multinational franchises along similar lines to Mcdonalds and Kentucky Fried Chicken with their ultimate goal being profit and not your health.

Now why do we promote this long known simple herbal beverage, tea? Because, in the last decades, in quite a few international longevity conferences and scientific seminars I have attended, tea, especially green tea, has been singled out as a unique herb carrying quite a few plant polyphenolic compounds that are protective of our body. Tea has been regarded as the best source of polyphenols and carotenoids while its caffeine content is low enough to induce no addiction. It is just mildly stimulating to the brain and muscles, and has no harmful side-effects. Recent studies have found tea has powerful antioxidants (catechins) which are superior to vitamin E and C in terms of their health benefits. At the same time two cups of green tea contain as much vitamin C as one glass of orange juice.

Here we better clear up the difference of current types of tea leaves for you to select the most suitable one to suit your taste:

There are only two kinds of tea plants that are commercially important – the Chinese variety and the Assam variety. From these, only the tips and young leaves are hand-picked and turned into the green and the black tea as the most popular tea leaves capable of improving our health. The rest like oolong and herbal/scented tea have been produced for local consumption and/or individual preference only.

Green tea

This beverage has a wide range of formidable catechins that according to a 1994 study protect the body against cancer especially oesophageal cancer (a common type of cancer among the Chinese) with up to a sixty per cent reduction of incidence among tea drinkers in Shanghai. Another study in Japan has demonstrated a forty-five per cent reduction of the incidence of lung cancer in tea-drinking smokers. Japan has a high smoking rate and yet a low lung cancer rate, so this is deemed altogether a most impressive finding.

In some American and Japanese studies on lab animals, it has been demonstrated that green tea fed to rodents protects them against all stages of cancers (initiation, promotion and progression), which is all attributed to the polyphenols it contains, as one of its catechins has been found to have special talent to block an enzyme called urokinase which is secreted by cancer cells in their attempt to open the door to invade cells and tissues.

The incredible potent polyphenol catechins in green tea have also been shown to lower cholesterols and reduce stroke, perhaps due to the ability of the catechins to reduce the stickiness of platelets – as the build-up of sticky platelets in some medical conditions can form blood clots (thrombus) which enter into circulation in the brain.

The tips and young leaves of green tea, after being picked, will usually be quickly sun dried and steamed to preserve their goodness, without fermentation, before being lightly pan-fried and vacuum-packed for export. This minimal processing appears to be the best way to preserve almost all the polyphenolics, carotenoids and antioxidants. I would also recommend that consumers store the whole package or the tin in the freezing compartment until it is ready to be used, and return the tin to the freezer after use each time, to make sure the goodness is not lost due to oxidisation. Of course, you store the good green tea leaves in the freezer only if you are not a regular tea drinker.

In one of my medical tours to China, our team took a detour to Han Zhow to visit the biggest producer of *Dragon Well*, the most famed and expensive green tea in the world. We were fortunate to have the opportunity to witness how it was minimally processed and carefully handled, while the head supervisor told us a light-hearted tale about the famed Soo Zhow girls whose beauty is attributed to their regular imbibing of the famous tea which helps nourish their fair skin and infuse energy into their facial features and bodily movements. They are also known to wash their face with *Dragon Well* tea and chew the leaves as well. A handy beauty tip!

Black tea
This comes from the same sort of leaf but it is handled very differently. The leaves are heated until they are withered, then crushed to allow oxidisation until their black colour is achieved. The fermentation process is kept going till the time it is brewed The end product is black, fine and crushed, but more aromatic with some flavour.

However, due to all this processing, the black tea has lost a great deal of its polyphenols and carotenoids. Compared with unfermented green tea which is estimated to contain about thirty per cent of those phenolics in its dry weight, the black tea is estimated to have lost about eighty per cent of them. So a better flavour is traded for fewer health benefits.

In general, black tea, packaged in a wide variety of ways, such as in teabags and bottled tea, is favoured by Westerners who often add milk and sugar to their individual taste.

Tip for a good brew of tea
One word about the art of brewing tea. The correct way is to warm up the teapot (far better than using just the cup) with boiled clean water (preferably filtered), empty half to one

teaspoon of vacuum-packed tea leaves into the cleaned pot and pour boiled hot water which has cooled to about seventy to eighty degrees in temperature. Wait for about fifteen to twenty minutes for the goodies of the tea leaves to infuse turning the water to light amber or pale green before you sip. You should be able to smell the subtle scent of the green tea if all the steps are followed properly.

he reason why the water temperature should not be too hot is to avoid scorching the leaves so that less tannin is infused to avoid giving the tea a butter taste. Also, the tea can be repeatedly brewed several times before most of the amino acids, polyphenols and carotenoids in the tea leaves become exhausted. The tea leaves can then be composted, leaving no waste.

Oils, the bad and the good

As you would recall from the beginning of this chapter, there are three major classes of macronutrients consisting of carbohydrates, proteins and fatty acids. Each one of them generates heat and energy when metabolised by your body, but to a different degree – by themselves the fatty acids (fats and oils) can produce twice as much energy in calories as carbs and proteins.

There are over forty varieties of fatty acids, but only three of them are important in the production of the hormones and enzymes your body needs to function and remain healthy. They are omega 3, omega 6 and linoleum acid which are called Essential Fatty Acids (EFA), or polyunsaturated fatty acids (PUFA) and can be obtained only from a small number of foods; while other non-essential fatty acids (NEFA) are available from most of the foods we ingest. NEFA usually just serves as fuel for your body to burn, thereby transforming it into heat and energy.

But before we look at the best ones for your health, we should look at the bad and harmful oils and why you should avoid them.

Dr Joseph Cheung

Fats to avoid

There are a few types of fats we call them 'bad fats'. Some come from vegetables including trans fat, palm oil, corn oil and coconut oil. Others come from animal products such as whole milk, cream, cheese, butter and fatty meats. These are saturated fats which turn solid at room temperature. After digestion they are transported to the liver which manufactures bad cholesterol (LDL type) and reduces your good cholesterol (HDL). LDL has been widely researched and proven to come from saturated fats. These infiltrate the blood vessel walls, where they slowly and steadily build up cholesterol plaques causing oxidative damage which will damage the heart in one of two ways. It may cause the artery to burst one day, and thereby cause an acute heart attack – this is nowadays recognised as the most common mode of cardiac emergency. Alternately, it can continue to fill up the major artery and block off the blood supply to the heart which may lead to a heart attack when there is some kind of extra exertion, like when the victim attempts to run after the bus, or hurries up a flight of stairs. So you are wise to keep your consumption of animal products and all the 'bad oils' as low as possible, or even near zero if your doctor tells you that your LDL is too high. Now let's look at all the bad fats we need to avoid:

Trans-fat is not found in nature, and didn't exist until its invention in 1900, but now takes up to six per cent of the market. It is produced by partially hydrogenating vegetable oil to become solid like margarine and vegetable shortening. This partial hydrogenation can stabilise the vegetable oil to make the products more solid and remain better preserved for commercial advantage. However, the chemical structure of trans-fat has been changed in such a way as to make it extremely harmful. Ingesting it regularly can lead to heart attack, stroke and NIDDM. It was recently banned by the FDA in the USA which forbids commercial manufacturers from adding any such trans-fat to any product. When you are shopping in supermarkets, you will notice most of the product will have displayed '0' against trans-fat unless the amount is minimal enough to be allowed by the FDA or the TGA in Australia).

In a 1993 one of the biggest, longest running studies ever conducted in US medical history – the Harvard Nurses' Study – with a total number of subjects of about 85,000, found that those who consumed the most margarine had a sixty-six per cent higher risk of heart disease than those who consumed a low amount of margarine. That is quite a convincing statistics but it does not come as a surprise because trans-fat has been found to give you a double whammy by raising your LDL (the bad cholesterol) while at the same time it reduces your HDL (the good cholesterol). Clearly even butter is better for you than those trans-fats!

In regard to Palm oil – this bad oil often hides under the name 'vegetable oil,' 'edible vegetable oil', or is purposely mixed among dozens of other obscure ingredients or co-ingredients, with the purpose of discouraging customers from checking the details. But you can be sure that most of the snacks, biscuits, pastry, sausages, cakes etc produced in Malaysia, Taiwan and China contain palm oil because it is mass produced in Indonesia and Malaysia and is much less expensive than good quality oils like Olive oil and peanut oil. The problem with palm oil is that it contains no less than fifty per cent saturated fat which if consumed in significant quantities could easily lead to you becoming a victim of CVD.

So it is CRUCIAL to check the ingredients of your supermarket groceries, making doubly sure you avoid 'trans-fat, partially hydrogenated fat, margarine, palm oil, corn oil and coconut oil'. Check your own fridge, if you can find any of the above fat products, throw them out. Use more healthy spreads for your children's sandwiches – recommended is tahini spread, almond butter spread, pickled paste, lemon butter spread, avocado, peanut butter, or even plain butter is to be preferred as long as you realise frequent and over-use can harm your CVS. I try to avoid attacking 'butter and milk'-they are the sacred cows in the western world and even many developing countries.

Omega 3

The first choice for good oils are the polyunsaturated Omega 3 fats in fish. According to Andrew Stoll, the Director of the psychiatry research lab at Harvard Medical school, Omega 3s are essential for mental health with remarkable anti-depressant powers, and they also enhance mood, memory and concentration, while monounsaturated vegetable and nut oils such as olive oils, peanut oils, rice bran oils are best for cooking.

Natural fat and oil from marine animals are mostly good oil with plenty of polyunsaturated omega 3 oil which keeps the fish and seals and polar bears healthy with good circulation even in the icy cold environment of the sea.

The Omega 3 polyunsaturated oils from fish are DHA (docosahexaenoic acid) and EPA (eicosapentaenoic acid), essential for the healthy development of the brain and the eyes in children, in addition to their anti-inflammatory actions for many conditions like rheumatoid arthritis, ulcerative colitis, asthma, and many other inflammatory diseases. When buying fish, make sure you go for small varieties like sardines, mackerel etc and avoid big fish like tuna and sword fish as big fish often contain more heavy metals such as mercury. To be on the safe side, talk to your doctor about having a blood test for heavy metals.

Omega 6

Furthermore, the Omega 6 oils found in canola oils, sunflower seed oil, walnut oils, are good for cooking. All are guaranteed good oils protective to your CVS and improve your immune system and health.

Professor Colin Campbell strongly believes that plant nutrition is far superior to animal protein and products in regard to prevention of CVD diseases, even in advanced stages. He gave some examples of world class athletes like iron man Dave Scott and track star Carl Lewi who reckon they have performed better on plant-based food than on animal-based.

To survive in this world of culinary wonders, most of us would prefer to have our dinner cooked. But the cooking methods have evolved a great deal since ancient time, to now we have at least eight to ten ways to prepare your dinner in European cuisine as represented by the French and the Italian style, while the Chinese has invented a dazzling thirty-six ways to cook your dinner.

Most cuisine requires good oils to cook quickly, to prepare the spice, herbs and condiments to bring their best flavour and aroma, as typically done in the Chinese stir-fry. Only the following methods use no oil at all – they use the water as medium or sheer heat or fire instead of oil, as in boiling, steaming and roasting (including BBQ).

The good oils are usually plant-based oils, with the best ones being olive oil, canola oil, grape-seed oil, rice-bran oil, sunflower seed oil, sesame oil, peanut oil, avocado oil, walnut oil and macadamia oil.

But the choice of the above oils depends on the type of cooking and ingredients, because they are somewhat different in their characteristics.

Olive Oil

For topping and salad dressing, olive oil, particularly the cold-pressed extra virgin kind is a safe choice for the European style, but sesame oil is preferred for Chinese cuisine for extra flavour. You can try others like walnut oil or avocado oil for more subtle flavour. Some cooking oils now have already infused different spices such as chilli, cinnamon, basil and other condiments for variety if you don't mind the spice sometimes being overbearing.

For stir-fry dishes, often you have to heat up the oil to a higher degree before you put in the spice and herbs to bring out the aroma and to seal the flavour of the meaty stuff that follows, then you have to make sure not to turn up the heat too high if you use olive oil because its smoke point (the temperature at which it begins to smoke) is only up to 200 C. Over-heating can alter the nature of the oil to change, in some part, to unhealthy trans oil. In Australia, we are fortunate to have a very reliable olive oil local producer – the Cobram estate in Victoria which has cultivated thousands of olive trees over the last twenty odd years, producing cold-pressed extra-virgin olive oils of excellent quality with price tags comparable to those imports from Mediterranean regions. As Australian, particularly in this Covid-19 pandemic, what better choice can you pick than buying good local products that are the freshest and the healthiest, indirectly you are also helping the local economy while enjoying your dinner done with quality extra virgin oils.

Rice-bran oil

For deep frying and high-heat cooking, is a better and safer choice than olive oil as it has a higher smoking point to 275-300 C. Some rice-bran oil even has an added plant steroid and vitamin E to provide more nutritional benefits. Always shop for a good brand that has all the good points of the oil listed.

Grape-seed oil

This is another good oil worth some attention. It is the by-product of the wine-making industry. Unfortunately, there is not much research on this oil, but it cannot be anything less than a promising powerful antioxidant health product containing many unravelled polyphenols, judging by the fact that resveratrol – the first polyphenol that activates our longevity gene – is the extract from grape skin/seed of distressed Pinot noir grapes. I have often used it myself for stir-fry and found its higher smoke point good to rely on as long as I watch that the gas fire is not turned too high. For home cooking, there is no point in using high heat anyway.

Peanut oil

This is a traditional oil used by the Chinese for several thousand years. But because of the more expensive price tag, it tends to be ignored by take-away shops and smaller cheap-eat set ups where you have no idea what sort of "vegetable" oils are being used. So recently I grab hold of a Chinese chef of thirty years' experience to get some insight. His view is that there cannot be much difference in the choice because in stir-frying, a small amount of peanut oil seems to do just as good job as cheaper oils which you need to pour more of. Well, think about it – a good point.

Proteins from Fish and Marine Animals

Here we come to the most important macronutrient that is required by every single one of the more than three trillion cells of the body. They are the building blocks of every living organism from the simplest single-cell living yeast to the most complex mammals like us. Proteins are the core components of your cells from the protective cellular wall to the central commanding nucleus containing all your genetic materials in the double helix, and thousands of enzymes interacting in the fierce intracellular complex of metabolic reactions. In reality, your body cannot afford to run out of proteins – they cannot be replaced by carbs or fatty acids.

Proteins are formed by amino acids – the basic organic chemicals in plants and animals. When you eat, the proteins in the food are broken down to the basic amino acids and absorbed into the blood. At any one time there can be over twenty different sorts of amino acids produced in the blood after digestion which will be transported to the liver and to all parts of the body for cellular metabolic use.

It is well established that plants foods, with their phytonutrients, are healthy, but they have one minor drawback which is that, except for soybeans, they do not contain nine of the essential amino acids which you have to obtain from animals (land or marine). But if you are fond of soybeans and its products, it will not be much of a problem because soybeans not only contain thirty-eight per cent protein, but they can also provide all nine essential amino acids we need. All the present-day soy products including tofu, soy milk and soy dessert are available at a very affordable price, and they are very wholesome too. Many people are not aware of the fact that the calcium content in soy milk in an average three hundred milligrams per serve, is practically the same as that found in cow's milk, yet without the risk of higher LDL to worry about.

Plant proteins are usually found concentrated in legumes, and in all kind of nuts and seeds. Marine animals such as fish, prawns and lobsters has been for a long time strongly recommended as the most healthy protein for our CVS, in contrast to land animals whose meat is liable to be contaminated with pesticides, chemicals and hormones to speed up meat production. Free-range chickens which are now readily available at butchers and supermarkets are always better than battery chickens. Their meat is leaner and tastier and gives you less LDL, which makes it well worth the extra dollar.

However, you still have to watch for pitfalls when buying fish meat. You have two choices – buy from the supermarket's fish/meat section, or a well-run fish shop. In general, it is easier to access a supermarket – there has to be one near where you live and these are usually managed reasonably well. But a fish monger is not easy to find unless you are close to a more populated suburb/town. Sometimes it is worthwhile to drive a few more miles to a good fish shop as you will find the quality and the variety of fish and seafood are superior to what you can find in a supermarket, even though usually it is more crowded and full of excitement from high spirited shoppers.

Now you also have to be aware that not all fish is equal in its health value: some are more meaty and muscular like swordfish from the deep sea, some might have more fine bones that could cause trouble in children. Some are imported from overseas countries like Vietnam, Thailand and you should try to avoid buying them (because we are not sure whether the fish was caught in heavily polluted water near industrial area, and how hygienic the products were packed and transported all the way to Australia. In short, those fish may be cheaper but carry higher risk as food. Possibly due to pollution, lesser strict inspection and quality control the fattier or oilier varieties are what you should aim for.

For a long time, scientists and researchers have found that fatty fish contain the most healthy omega 3 polyunsaturated oils which have been proven time and time again sine late 1980s to be protective against breast, prostate and colorectal cancers. A big study by British scientists, which compared cancer rates in twenty-four European countries, concluded that cancer rates rose with eating more land animal meat and fat, but decreased when more fish and fish oils were consumed.

Another study done in Finland, interestingly, discovered the fish oils level was much higher in women with only breast tumour, but lower in women with breast cancer. That can be translated as that the higher level of fish oil ingestion appeared to be protecting the women against their tumour developing into cancer.

Other surveys appeared to show a parallel incidence for men's prostate cancers.

The following list of fatty fish and other common varieties serves only as a guide, and you will have to experiment for yourself to find what suits your individual taste:

Fatty fish
- sardines
- herring
- mackerel
- salmon
- trout

- tuna
- pilchards
- Murray cod
- perch

Other varieties

- rock ling
- bream
- sea perch
- John Dory
- swordfish
- barramundi
- whiting
- snapper
- sole
- flounder
- trevally
- leather jacket

There are two more unusual types of food I would recommend though not readily available even at the fish market (the extremely popular Sydney's fish market, should be the first one Sydneysiders head to as it has a huge range of fish, king crabs, lobsters, sea-urchins etc) but be prepared to get there early before mid-day to avoid huge crowds pouring out from tourist buses all clamouring and fighting to get to the counters to get plate after plate of seafood, infusing the atmosphere with aroma that seems to instantly pump up your appetite. Though it isn't like that if there is a lockdown.

Crocodile

The more unusual type of food I have in mind is crocodile meat and frog meat. Crocodiles are semi-aquatic reptiles many of whom are confined to fresh-water environments and frogs are amphibians who also live in rivers and lakes. Crocodile meat, like the meat of other reptiles, such as goannas and snakes, tastes soft and succulent and is often compared to chicken, so it is best cut into slices, stir-fried with garlic and ginger and combined with your favourite vegies.

This dish is as commonly available at seaside restaurants in northern Queensland towns like Cairns and Townsville as those beautifully cooked and tender spring lamb are in New Zealand. Frog legs, on the other hand, have been a famed French cuisine for many years because of their delicate and tasty texture which makes them highly sought after by the French gourmets. But frog legs are no less popular either among Chinese gourmets in Hong Kong and Kwang Zhow (Canton), where they are often presented as an entrée at a banquet.

Tips on buying fish

Always check, if buying whole fish, the eyeball should be as transparent as possible, the gill should be bright red and the flesh firm to touch. For busy working couples, perhaps a better way is to buy fish fillet or cutlet to save much work in your preparation to cook them. When cooking seafood, never forget to add garlic, ginger, spring onion, some coriander leaves and a liberal amount of cold-pressed extra virgin oil, (and I usually like to splash some sesame oil to add more aroma to a complete garnish of this healthy food).

A note of warning on allergies

Now we are more than happy to recommend a meal of fresh fish for everybody, at least two to three times a week, if possible, unless you are considering being more adventurous with sea food and want to try the more luxurious, more expensive seafoods like prawns and lobsters, scallops, and oysters, sea cucumbers and so forth. But if you do, you must make sure you are NOT allergic to any of them, particularly prawns. Prawn allergy may be more common than you might imagine.

Once, when I was acting as a locum near Maitland in NSW, Australia, my wife and I invited another locum, Dr M, to come home for dinner so we could get to know each other better. As good hosts, we liked to prepare some good food for our guest. In those days in the sixties, seafood was rather expensive, but we were fortunate to spot some green (uncooked) prawns which would enable us to prepare some top cuisine, stir-fried with gingers and spring onions. We were rubbing our hands in glee when we could smell the wonderful aroma of fried prawns streaming out of the kitchen. Suddenly, I noticed our guest's face dropped and he looked unwell, muttering, 'Sorry Joe, I forgot to tell you that I am allergic to prawns since I ate some bad ones years ago. It has really put me off since.' He couldn't even stay in the room and had to go home!

Another time in Melbourne, Victoria, we were at a regular gourmet dinner meeting where a well-established dentist was joining us. Being a friend of one of our dentist friends, he was most welcome to share the sumptuous eight-course dinner we always have. This dentist, Dr Y, appeared to be exceptionally cautious. He personally talked to the waiter and even the chef and checked every course of dish. Then his wife finally burst out, 'You know what he is doing? He is trying to find out if any prawn ingredient or even juice/sauce/stock with trace of prawn in it. My husband is EXTREMELY allergic to prawns'. And she went on to explain that she had used the term 'extremely' with good reason because, she said, her husband had had a few times been ambulanced to hospital when he had collapsed after eating nothing spectacular other than some soup (suspected to have prawns for added flavour) or prawn-juice contaminated cuisine. Even just trace of it! We jokingly suggested that he should carry his own personalised adrenaline injection in his pocket.

Meat from Land Animals

Pork, beef and lamb

In countries like North America, Australia, New Zealand and UK, meat is a big part of the diet and beef steaks and lamb chops reign supreme at the dinner, while vegetables used to be treated as farmer's tucker, not worth a second helping. In fact some people are used to having meat from mammals three times a day, like bacon or sausages for breakfast, ham or canned meat for lunch, then steak or chops for dinner.

According to Professor Fontana, in a 2016 survey, Americans top the world in devouring ninety-seven kilos of red meat (and top the world in MI) followed by Australians consuming ninety-five kilos, and Argentinians sixty-nine kilos. However, Fontana has also noted that since 1961 red meat consumption has gone up fifteen times in China, and fourfold in Brazil. And it is almost predictable that MI and cancer rate would have crept up, even though slowly, if a survey is to be conducted soon. His statistics has greatly shocked me, but I agree with his conclusions absolutely, because it's just a straightforward logic that more red meat means higher LDL cholesterol and an increased incidence of heart attacks.

People not aware of the risk of cancer associated with the consumption of red meat which is regarded by WHO as a Group two carcinogen (processed meat being a Group one carcinogen) as well as its association with a high risk of CVD, obesity and NIDDM. Now red meat has also been found to produce a metabolite in the gut called TMAO which causes the above chronic medical conditions. Those Sunday BBQs, if the meat is over cooked and burnt, can produce in addition to the usual risks, a high concentration of amines and compounds which are potent mutagenic molecules and harmful to your DNA. Also, Fontana points out that red meat is rich in iron (heme) which on being broken down in the gut will generate N-nitroso compounds which are highly carcinogenic too. So best to steer away from not only processed meat, but also red meat in general, for the sake of your health and longevity.

The red-meat trend is understandable because Europeans and Westerners are brought up in dairy-farming environments where there are grassy paddocks and hills. They have become dependent on everything from dairy farming, and have been taught, one might say 'brain washed', that cow's milk contain lots of calcium and proteins to make children's bones strong once children are weaned. They are further encouraged to believe that beef and other animal meat is the best source of protein to help build strong muscles and afford plenty of energy to play and run faster. And, of course, it must be admitted that steaks and chops, when fried or grilled, do give out an appetising aroma because of the searing effect of fire on meat protein and juice.

So traditionally, most workers come home expecting to have meat for dinner, perhaps with cheese and a glass of cow's milk, followed by a rich desert topped with chocolate syrup covered ice cream (made of milk, butter and vegetable shortening). Next morning, the breakfast is mostly dairy foods like milk, cheese, bread spread with thick butter and jam, maybe bacon and egg when something "heartier" is desired. In the not-so-recent past, many relished a classical British breakfast of 'bacon and eggs' which made them feel satisfied that they had looked after their tummy before a hard day's work.

For centuries, no one suspected the link between early death from heart attack and dairy food and land-animal meat. But with the publication of modern demographic surveys, death statistics and studies from many cardiac and cancer research centres at reputable universities and institutes the evidence has mounted up overwhelmingly as to what is really going on. The following findings represent a small sampling of what has been discovered:

In 1981, two well-known British epidemiologists, Richard Doll and Richard Peto, were commissioned by the US Congress to investigate the cause of high cardiac death rate in the US. The report presented to the US Congress simply pointed out that the major culprits were cigarette smoking and diet. They put the blame squarely on the consumption of excessive animal meat and unhealthy fatty food, and the recommended countermeasures were to reduce animal meat consumption while increasing the amount of vegetables and fruits. This early study has been vindicated by many since.

In 2003, a comprehensive survey in the US showing the top eighteen causes of death in the US – listed CVD as number one. It was responsible for twenty-eight per cent of all deaths, which was estimated as being seventeen times higher than the rate in China. That is three thousand deaths from heart attack per day which has now reduced to two thousand only due to the introduction of new life-saving cardiac procedures like stenting, CABG and pacemakers etc.

In Australia, famed internationally for its impressive image of healthy, bronzed lifesavers patrolling Bondi beach, the landscape does not look that rosy either. Just three years ago a warning was issued by the National Heart Foundation on Father's Day that reminded people to check their heart due to a recent statistic which showed that over ten thousand Australians had perished from heart attack in the previous year.

The key problem remains the elevated LDL. This rogue cholesterol has been recognised for decades by researchers and cardiologists as the culprit. It builds up in the coronary arterial wall, causing damage by oxidising radicals on one hand, but also by starting to damage and destabilize the endothelium (the inner lining of the artery) and causing heart attack without warning. This is the most common way of heart attacks presents. I myself observed it in my lifetime of medical consulting and the two hundred-plus autopsies I took part in at the Ottawa General Hospital in Canada.

So how many people have high cholesterol levels in the general population? According to surveys carried out between 1980-2000, about fifty per cent of Australians according to Professor A Tonkins of the National Heart Foundation, and from forty to forty-eight per cent by the reckoning of other experts.

Yet only about fifteen per cent of Americans were found to have abnormal levels in the 2013 survey conducted by the American Heart Association. That did not seem to tally well with their high death rate from MI (up to twenty-eight per cent). One of the reasons could be the different standard of what is 'high'; the other reason could be that Americans have headed the wake-up call to Americans to keep up their lipid lowering medication after Bill Clinton's quadruple by-pass.

In recent years, many internationally well-known cardiologists and researchers have repeatedly pointed out that land animal meats, dairy and unhealthy cooking oils have been found to increase your LDL, give you higher homocysteine (one of the triggers for heart attack), more hormones to give you hormone-dependent cancers, more toxins from insecticides, weed-killers spray, DDT, PCB contaminated milk, organochlorine metabolites (found in one hundred per cent of autopsy samples). All this clear data has been collected by Professor C. Campbell, Dr Gaynor, Professor J Kahn and Professor D Sinclair mong others.

Cancer is rated the number two killer in the US: responsible for twenty-three per cent of all death. The most common types are breast, lung, CRC (colon-rectal) and prostate. The breast-cancer death rate, in Japan, where veggies and fish are staples rather than meat and dairy, is reported to be about six per one hundred thousand as compared to over twenty-two per one hundred thousand in the US. The breast cancer rate has also been favourably low in China.

Clearly the big factor between the high cancer rate in the US and the low cancer rate in Japan and China is that the caloric intake of protein among Americans is eighty per cent animal protein as China and all centenarian regions inhabitants only consume ten per cent (Okinawa nine per cent) from animal protein with the rest coming from plant proteins like legumes and soybeans. In fact, Dr A Weil, an experienced nutritionist, strongly promotes soybeans as the best food for most of the proteins we need. The reason, as we have described in previous chapters, is that soybeans are the only legume that contain all the essential amino acids found in animal meat, and, what's more, they are loaded with phytohormones and polyphenols that are protective of your body against hormone-dependent cancers such as breast, prostate, CRC and pancreatic.

Without further introduction, most of you, I am pretty sure, would have no fuss at all about animal meats that you can see displayed in any butcher shops, supermarkets. But there are a few, including fowl, that seem to offer you some nutritional value and are less harmful and deserve being mentioned for the sake of completeness for this 'meaty' section:

Quail and pigeon
Both present healthy lean meat if prepared and roasted properly. Both are semi-gourmet fair that's worth an occasional trial as some people find their unusual texture and taste exquisite.

Rabbit, kangaroo and venison
All available on the market. All these are very lean and nutritious. Not much aroma but very meaty flavour after a good stir-fry with suitable spices, condiments and plenty of extra-virgin olive oil. New Zealand is probably the best place for venison, as the herd of deer are kept in special farms in a natural environment and at just the right climate.

I have had such favourable experience on some succulent venison and spring lamb at a feast in Christchurch during our family tour to celebrate our two adult children entering the medical faculty. This was a few years before the devastating earthquake that toppled many historic churches and killed many people. We found quite a few excellent restaurants for our culinary venture. The wonderfully fulfilling aromatic dishes are remembered by my tastebuds until today.

Other meat like pork, beef and lamb are something that you should regard as a last resort for your proteins, keeping in mind that they only give you excess LDL, harmful fatty acids, higher chance for cancers, and make you put on weight too.

If you prefer a greener healthier environment, you should all the more reduce the animal type of protein because all these land animals damage and pollute the environment. So, for that matter do wild pigs, bulls, camels and brumbies (there are estimated to be about fourteen thousand of these wild horses running wild in the Mt Kosciuszko National Park, where they damage the vegetation, the bush and possibly some endangered species of wild flowers). They should be culled systematically to protect the delicate ecosystems. Even iconic animals like the kangaroo need to be and have been culled regularly to preserve the vegetation.

Chapter Eight: The Real Fountain of Youth

As you may recall from an earlier chapter, in 1513, over five hundred years ago, the Spanish explorer Ponce De Leon set out to look for the fabled Fountain of Youth along the coast of Florida. Of course, he found nothing of the kind, but left a legacy for inquisitive minds to keep searching, exploring, theorising, studying and experimenting at numerous reputable research centres, universities and medical institutes of the global community.

During the time of the writing and preparation of this book for publication, Covid-19 has raged. It is the most significant pandemic since the Spanish flu epidemic which wiped out seventeen million people and the worst in the living memory of anyone alive today. As everybody knows, the global economy has been severely devastated due to the frequently repeated lock-downs of most businesses and curtailed daily activities of the general public including international travel, intranational commuter traffic and local shopping life. Many businesses and companies have been forced to close down or have gone out of business.

Australia has been most unfortunate to be hit with a double whammy. Firstly, the horrific bushfire 2019-2020 was uncontrollable and caused over 10 million hectares of bushland completely torched, thirty-three lives lost, and over three thousand homes destroyed. Then it was immediately followed by the Covid-19 pandemic, the international shut down of borders and even interstate ones as well, which was absolutely illogical and often unnecessary, and has become a long running battle between state premiers at every morning's news briefings on TV. The public was sick of it because of the great inconvenience and frustration, particularly for the border residents. Can you imagine that within twenty-four hours (at times shorter notice) you have to cancel all your travel arrangements or face two weeks' quarantine in a hotel at your own expense whenever a few cases have been picked up in one state causing some premiers to press the panic button. They have a miserably scanty idea of how many hours people need to rush back to their own home from another state, only to have to face another hurdle of checking their ID at the border after driving for hours and joining the long queue of home-bound traffic.

One good thing this pandemic has brought us is that people now have become smarter and can see which premier has more common-sense and which one is highly strung and has a knee jerk reaction that can send the entire state and its prosperity into a nose-dive. Well, like everything else in life, not much you can do with unfriendly or uncooperative neighbours except to keep up daily bickering, sparring and arguing.

However, Australia is still a lucky country because of its relatively isolated geographic position as a natural defence against uncontrolled people traffic across the national border as if a floodgate had been installed and shut tight. The latest statistics of Covid-19 both in the world, the USA, and Australia (up to the fourteen of July 2022), presents to us a very interesting picture of the huge contrast of devastation under different management as shown below :

Secrets of Longevity

Worldwide	total positive cases	total number of deaths
	559 million	6.36 million
USA	89.1 million	1.02 million
Australia	8.56 million	10385

Now that the wretched 2020 is long gone and soon be relegated to the back of our mind, 2021 already heralded in exciting news that there are at least four to five new vaccines to counteract against the covid-19. With the vaccination being effectively carried out the boarders have finally been opened and international travel is once more a possibility.

So the future, although not quite rosy, is at least emerging a little bit of a lovely pink in the year 2022. In fact, because of the universal removal of border restrictions we have now witnessed a boom in travelling which resulted in chaotic scenes at most airports around the world with hundreds and thousands of travellers standing in long queue wanting to check in to fly out of the country for various purposes. Particularly during the school holidays, deeply frustrated travellers waited for hours due to the frequent cancellation of flights and long delays during processing before boarding. The airlines blame all these on shortage of administration staff, at luggage handlers, and even qualified air pilots. Shortage of skilled workers has been a universal reality in most businesses, small and large, due to the effects of Covid-19.

In the meantime, the versatile disease progresses relentlessly and has been detected to have mutated into variants of B4 and 5. The new strains have been found to be more infectious and more able to weakening the immunity of people who have had a third vaccination: the booster. So the health authorities in Australia have rushed to urge the public since mid-2022 to protect themselves again with more booster injections (a fourth), by wearing a mask in public places and keeping a distance from one another, once again.

Obviously, the war against tCovid-19 is not finished yet. Everyone needs be alert and to follow the rules to protect oneself and the community

Meanwhile, there is more good news for the future healthy global community as I believe we are now approaching closer to dipping our toe into the waters of the Fountain of Youth by practising the following list of essential good habits and activities, as much as you can, to push back ageing and chronic medical illnesses and give you a few more youthful years of healthy life, disease free, cancer free, worry free, yet filled with lively memories and happiness for the rest of your life.

The following recommendations in summary are the crystallised product of years of research, diligent study, hundreds of thousands of experiments and demographic surveys by brilliant global scientists, dedicated researchers, academics and government agencies. Most of the recommendations have been proven to work successfully not only on laboratory animals, but on humans as well, as quoted and reported on by many reputable medical journals.

Adopt and practise as many recommendations as you can, within your amiable lifestyle and individual preferences, but *do it regularly* and make it part of your new routine until it becomes habit. My intuition tells me that you could push back your ageing's advance and award yourself with quite a few extra years' in lifespan, healthier and happier.

In addition, remember that hereditary influence are not strong, and unlikely to be more than ten to fifteen per cent, while environmental good efforts to transform your lifestyle to a healthy one are the dominant and the most powerful force.

Regular Exercise

It has been known and proven that exercise is a kind of stress that stimulates your longevity gene (or vitality gene) – the sirtuins molecule to become more active in repairing any damage to your DNA and regulating your good genes to be more protective.

You just pick the type of exercise you like, such as hiking, slow or fast walking, jogging/running, or water sports like swimming and hydrotherapy exercises, cycling, ball games, even golfing and dancing. And if you don't feel strong enough, choose more gentle ones like dancing, walking, Tai Chi, or indoor freeform movements.

You can do them at home, on a balcony or football field, in the back yard or gym, … anywhere as long as you are in a healthy space, away from polluted air and the noisy crowd. Best to exercise with moderate intensity so that you feel comfortable, not out of breath and not dizzy, but with your heart beating faster, sweating a bit, and usually feeling more energy, with your whole body loosening up. The entire experience should leave you feeling happier. Contrary to some opinions, high intensity exercise has no additional benefit and may inflict more harm or damage to your body.

I generally swim three times a week and walk/jog three times a week, and I did so before carrying out my regular day of medical consultation, for forty odd years, until I retired in 2020 at the age of eighty-five – still rather young compared to Okinawa's centenarian, but deemed 'too old' by the bureaucratic medical board to take care of my patients, even though none of the board members are or have been a family doctor – not unlike a one-sided judgement offered by two blind men on an elephant. Someone has aptly dubbed it the 'armchair medical board' – but they seem to be specialists good in finding fault with hard-working GPs and being, at times, absolutely intolerant of even minor deviation from their set of official guidelines (which do not seem to have sufficient input from GPs) in the name of 'protecting the public's health'. Recently a powerful movement has been underway by a group of doctors and specialists who in the past have suffered at the hands of the medical board to challenge the unfair and unnecessary judgements by the board, with an ultimate proposal to the government/senate to radically reform the medical board. When our voice is getting louder and roaring, the government will listen. About time, I think.

My experience with regular exercise has always been enjoyable and even blissful. And if you keep it up in a good rhythm for years, you may not need Calorie Restriction to live longer.

Daily stretching, loosening up

Any time after spending an hour or so, it is advisable to get up from your office chair, to stretch your body, your arms and shoulders, walk a few minutes, to avoid poor posture induced chronic low back pain – one of the commonest complains and back conditions seen in general medical practice. It invariably happens to sedentary office workers, accountants, doctors, typists and taxi drivers. It will then, if you don't take notice and prevent it, develop into all different forms of lumber spine damage and progressively become harder to restore to normal. So regular stretching and exercise will help.

Eat More Greens and Less meat and dairy

This should be one of your most vital changes of habit and a fundamental practise to protect your body and extend your life.

As described in detail in the last chapter on Green Power, most vegetables, fruits etc. are loaded with vitamins, minerals and polyphenols to provide us with macro- and micro-nutrients – the phytonutrients including many enzymes and chemicals whose potential we are still not fully aware of. Nevertheless, some of the chemicals from grapes, green tea and soybeans have already been discovered to be capable of switching on our vitality genes and good genes, repairing our DNA to prolong our lives and protect us from more damage by viruses, bacteria, radiation and chemicals.

They may not be as tasty and appetising as roasted meat, BBQ and deep-fried chicken, but plants carry far fewer harmful chemicals, industrial poisons and harmful hormones that cause you to put on weight and become a diabetic, give you CVD and a much higher chance of getting cancer. The centenarian in China, Sardinia and Okinawa are perfect role models for all of us in the West – who have been consuming too much red meat and dairy – because those centenarians are healthier, have much less sickness, hardly any chronic illness, and a very low incidence of cancers of all sorts. Furthermore, their land, rivers and forests are not polluted by dairy farming and industrial chemicals.

Go for fatty fish for your animal proteins – for example Atlantic salmon, trout, sardines, barramundi, etc. all very fresh and tasty and protective to your heart.

Select good nutritious oils like cold-pressed extra-virgin olive oil and peanut oil. Avoid margarine, lard, hydrogenated oil, palm oil, coconut oil and dripping (saturated fat from fatty part of beef and lamb).

Calorie Restriction

CR is said to be the most consistent factor when it comes to the extension of lifespan. It has been advocated even as far back as Hippocrates' time – easily over two thousand years ago. It has been proven time and time again in experiment on lab animals including fruit flies, worms and rodents. Most of the time scientists are pretty impressed by their lifespan extension of up to fifty per cent.

However, as you can imagine, CR is almost like starving – restricting your food, and it appears the extra years you may gain are in direct proportion to the amount of food you eat less. It is difficult, to say the least, for any human to survive on restricted potions when they are feeling hungry and need fuel to give them energy and heat. Hence, you have to weigh the benefits of living extra years against the sufferings of hunger before you should wade into this lifestyle.

The good news is that recently some researchers have become convinced that a different form of CR could still help you to gain more years of life – this is the so-called intermittent CR. In other words, you can skip a meal now and then, or have a day without food, or a block of days per month or per year in which you eat less. This way is more flexible and tolerable and can be tried out by anyone, particularly overweight sedentary workers.

We can have a look at the lifestyle of most centenarians in China and Okinawa who impressed investigating scientists with their habit of eating only until they are eighty per cent full – another form of CR that can be easily tried.

Learn How to Relax and Sleep Well

The world we inhabit nowadays is full of unpleasant noises: rumbling traffic, honking horns, construction sounds, screeches, sirens and high-pitched irritating voices, sometimes even screams. Driving in your car to work you are still not entirely shielded from those unwanted noises in the cities and busy shopping centres which often over stimulate your nervous system, irritating your sensitive neurons.

In addition, you may have worries and problems in your office that might come back at night to haunt you. So, basically, when all these little irritations add up, your muscles and system become tense which may not easily unwind.

No wonder over fifty per cent of people suffer from insomnia, tension headaches, migraine and mental health problems like depression and anxiety, etc. So how do you relax well before bedtime in order to get a sweet sleep? It's not easy unless you develop a good healthy lifestyle first, then try one or more than the following techniques:

Deep-breathing exercises

Using abdominal breathing instead of your chest. It is utilised by all practitioners of Tai Chi, martial arts, and by meditating Buddhist monks. It has a calming effect.

Meditation

This is just a simple method to concentrate on a word or a phrase, a kind of mindfulness, as long as you make it a habit or routine, a few minutes in a quiet corner, to re-train your mind to do what you want it to.

Tai Chi, Yoga, and other exercises

These practices are the secret formula used by Eastern practitioners to calm the mind and settle yourself when you are jittery, and soothe your irritable nerves. These days you should have no trouble finding them on/line. Short demonstration videos or discs can be bought cheaply. Practise them at home at your leisure.

Wonder Drugs

In Chapter Five, we mentioned at least five types of chemicals that have been intensely studied by Professor D Sinclair and found to contribute to our ability to fight off ageing by activating and reinforcing our vitality genes. Some are available on the market, either through the pharmacy, or by direct order on line:

Resveratrol

It is recommended to take from fifty milligrams up to one hundred and fifty milligrams per day with no unpleasant side effects reported, even at the larger dose. It directly switches on the longevity gene to protect your DNA, your genes and your immune system against damaging infection.

Metformin

This one, listed by WHO as one of the cheapest, most versatile chemicals yet with the lowest side effects. It is an oral anti-diabetic drug, but amazingly has been found capable of activating SIRT (the longevity gene) to help prolong life and inhibit cancer cell metabolism especially in breast cancer. It has been found to help women suffering PCOS (polycystic ovarian syndrome) to improve and regain their fertility – how amazing! It is also said to alleviate mental ill-health.

You still need a prescription from your doctor. Suggested dosage being two hundred and fifty milligrams to five hundred milligrams once or twice a day. Always start on a lower dose to see how you feel for a week or so, bearing in mind that most early NIDDM patients take five hundred milligrams, twice a day, at times up to one thousand milligrams twice a day.

Nicotinamide Adenosine Dinucleotide (or NAD)

This is another STAC (SIRT1 activating compound) capable of boosting all seven sirtuins in our cells and is used by over five hundred different enzymes in our body. It acts as fuel for the longevity genes too. So it is clearly a busy chemical, very much in demand when it comes to fighting the advance of ageing and all sorts of chronic illnesses and cancer.

Vitamin B3 turns into NAD in our bodies and also increases with regular exercise. NAD occurs naturally in some foods, notably easy way out is to buy its precursor, vitamin B3, is available online in Australia and New Zealand, and in the US, too, of course. fatty fish, avocado, broccoli, cabbage and others. Again, your

In addition, some other supplements are highly recommended as a harmless but powerful anti-oxidant and anti-inflammatory substance, the following two can be taken daily and all the time for auxiliary help as mentioned before: Green tea and Isotonix opc-3 (containing bilberry/grape seed/Pycnogenol).

Be connected, be part of the community

We have stressed this point time and time again, that we, *homo sapiens*, being social animals, have always had the desire to live close to each other – with your partner and off-spring as a family unit, to work together as a team to help each other in an enjoyable work environment, and gradually merge in larger groups to form a secure community in which every individual and every team helps one another as part of a modern township or regional centre. People tend to socialise with others sharing similar common interests and intelligent conversation where they can be emotionally and intellectually fulfilled, happier, with far less susceptibility to mental ill-health.

On the other hand, people who alienate themselves from their work mates and isolate themselves from their family and friends, are not much different from a lonely stray animal and are more prone to mental health issues like anxiety, depression and may even develop some form of psychosis. Therefore, you are strongly advised to socialise with your family, extended family and friends, and to join in on community activities, to attend religious services, and voluntary charity services. That is the best way to feel fulfilled and happy in your inner self. In other words, you simply move forward with the crowd, with your preferred purpose or target in mind, to enjoy your healthy, happy and longer life.

Habits to avoid

The following items are part of a healthy lifestyle which you should practise in order to reinforce the solid foundation from which you build up more energy and vitality for a stronger immune system and protection of your DNA and genetic materials due to stimulating more vigorous vitality genes:

Cigarette/tobacco smoking

Avoiding smoking is the best way to prevent their powerful carcinogens which may induce lung cancer (being aware of the four thousand chemicals you can inhale into your lungs). Those who contract this terrible disease will suffer in a very painful and debilitating, which is one of the main culprits singled out by Richard Doll to blame for the high death rate in the US during a survey in 1981. Every cigarette smoked could shorten your life by seven minutes.

Excessive alcohol consumption

Just observe the recommended limits of alcohol consumption described in an earlier chapter. Alcoholism will give you gastritis, liver damage and brain damage, even cancer of the liver or pancreas. Even a single drinking binge can result in severe damage and even death.

Drugs of addiction

All "party drugs" and "recreation drugs" are highly dangerous and powerfully addictive, particularly for younger persons ignorant of the dangers and the traps laid by drug peddlers. Somehow Australia has been a soft target by drug cartels from SEA and South America. In parallel with addictive gambling, once you are in, you are gone forever, no more healthy long life for you. In fact, no more life left in you.

The summing up

By seriously practising most or even all the major recommendations in this chapter, and making them your lifelong habits, your body and your immune system will have got the upper hand against most viruses, bacterial infections, high-risk cardiovascular diseases and many debilitating chronic diseases like asthma, diabetes, painful osteoarthritis, the dreaded Alzheimer disease, and many others.

Put simply: it just equates to a life with minimal pain and suffering, a life full of creative energy to contribute to society, a life of fulfillment and happiness shared with your family, relatives and friends, a life of enjoying the never-ending beauty of the sun, the moon, the blue sky and our incredibly magnificent Earth.

NOW, our final conclusion at this date and age is, for anyone interested in healthy ageing is that some extra years can be regained provided you adopt a healthy lifestyle for the rest of your life. You may ask when should we start? We would suggest AS SOON AS POSSIBLE, mindful that the life clock of biological changes and degeneration have already started ticking from the time of conception.

My routine
And lest you think this is all nice in theory, let me share with you the daily routine that has kept me fit and active up to my current age of eighty-seven – not bad considering I could have done somewhat better with my diet in my younger days

The daily routine of
Dr Joseph Cheung, OAM

- Morning – up 4:30 to 5:00
- Three mornings a week, swim freestyle fifty to sixty laps (in a twenty-five metre indoor pool) plus four laps of backstroke
- Walking/jogging alternate mornings, about forty-five minutes to an hour. (This means daily exercise, rarely missed a day (except for the Covid-19 years) for nearly forty years.)

- Breakfast – porridge with soy milk, or muesli with soy milk, a slice of multigrain, or rye, or sourdough bread, with non-dairy spread
- Often a piece of fruit.
- Medication

- 1 x 100mg cartia (asprin)
- 1x vit B3 500mg
- 250mg of Metformin
- 1x Co-Q 10 150mg

- Lunch – used to be just one home-made sandwich with tahini or almond paste spread, or canned sardine, plus a piece of fruit. Now after retirement, I have more time to cook brown rice or noodles or purple potatoes (no instant pre-packed ones) with vegies, sardines or tuna.
- Dinner – with my more packed full lunch, I tend to get on to a simple meal for dinner, such as some soup, some congee, or a small potion of left-over food or sweet potato (choose the purple flesh one)
- Medication
    - 250mg of metformin
    - Lipitor 20mg x 1
- Social dinner/feast gatherings – whenever, but try to eat less meat and only eighty per cent full.
- Religious attendance – only joined in recently, Sunday morning, still have to wait until Covid-19 rule relaxed

Note – since cutting down much land animal meat I have increased my greens/fruits even eating more at lunch, I have lost up to five kilos.

My recommended food pyramid

sweets
poultry
meat, eggs
fish and
seafood
herbs, spices, condiments

legumes, nuts seeds,
foods rich in calcium ad flavonoids:
soy products (tofu, soy milk etc.) fruits, avocado,
olive oils, omega 3 oils

vegetables in great variety
especially green leafy ones
whole grains, noodles, oats, Basmati and brown rice

| daily | 3 times a week | occassional if at all | seldom, best never |

drink tea daily if you like, alcohol in moderation,
and eat some dark chocolate on occassion

References and Selected Further Reading

Chapters two and three

Buettner, D, *The Blue Zones,* National Geographic, 2008.

Day, John D, and Jane Ann, LaPlante, M, *The Longevity Plan,* Harper Collins, 2017.

Esselstyn Jr, Caldwell B. *Prevent and Reverse Heart Disease,* Penguin Books, 2008.

Flanigan, R J, sawyer, K F, *Longevity Made Simple,* Williams Clarke Publishing, 2007

Hills, B, *The Island of the Ancients,* Murdoch Books, Crows Nest, 2008.

Wilcox, B J, Wilcox, D C, Suzuki, M, *The Okinawa Program,* Three Rivers Press, New York, 2001.

Chapter four

Cheung, J Y T, Total Health and Fitness Revolution, Possible Press, 2019.

Costello, P, The Costello Memoirs, Melbourne University Press, 2008.

Esselstyn, Jr, Caldwell, B, Prevent and Reverse Heart disease, Penguin Books, 2008.

Fontana, L, The Path to Longevity, Hardie Grant, 2020.

Gaynor, M, with Hickey, J, Cancer Prevention Program, Kensington books, 1999.

GP Update Handbook, Primary Care International, 2016.

Kahn, J K, *The Whole Heart Solution*, Reader's Digest, 2013.

Longmore, M, Wilkinson I, B, Rajagopalan, S, *Oxford Handbook of Clinical Medicine*, Oxford University Press, 2006.

Lundell, D, Nordstrom, T, R, *The Cure for heart Disease,* Heart Surgeon's Health Plan, LLC, 2007.

Maroon, J, *The Longevity Factor,* Atria, 2009.

Ornish, D, *Dr dean Ornish's Program for Reversing Heart disease,* Ballantine Books,1996.

Sinclair, D A, with LaPlante, M D, *Lifespan,* Thorson, London, 2019.

Taylor, J, B, *My Stroke of Insight*, Hodder & Stoughton,2008.

Wentz, M, *Invisible Miracles,* photocopies, 2000.

Woodruff, R, *Cancer Pain,* Asperula, Vic. Australia, 2013.

Chapter Five

Braun, L, Cohen, M, *Herbs and Natural Supplements,* Elsevier Mosby, Australia, 2005. Cheung, J, Y, T, *Total Health and Fitness Revolution,* Possible Press,2019.

Cheung, S C, *Chinese Medicinal Herbs of Hong Kong,* Commercial Press, Hong Kong, 1980.

Esselstyn Jr, Caldwell, 8, *Prevent and Reverse Heart Disease,* Penguin.

Fontana, L, *The Path to Longevity,* Hardie Grant Books, London, 2020.

MIMS, MIMS Australia, 2009

Sinclair, D, with La Plante, M, D, *Lifespan,* Thorson, London,2019.

Sydney Morning Herald, on Inquiries in Crown Sydney, various news articles published from January to February 2021.

Chapter six

Bolton, J, *The Room Where It Happened,* Simon & Schuster, NY, 2020.

Gate, B. *The Road Ahead*, Australian Print Group, 1995.

O'Brien, C, *Never Say Die,* Harper Collins, Australia, 2008.

Sinclair, D, with La Plante, M, D, *Lifespan,* Thorson, London, 2019.

Chapter seven

Braun, L, Cohen, M, *Herbs & Natural Supplements,* Elsevier Mosby,2005. Buettner, D, *The Blue Zones Kitchen,* National Geographic, 2019

Campbell, T C, with Campbell 11, T M, *The China Study,* Benbella Books, Texas, USA, 2005.

Cheung, J Y T, *Total Health and Fitness Revolution,* Possible Press,2019.

Day, J D, Day, J A, LaPlante, M, *Longevity Plan,*

Harper Collins, 2017.

Dunlop, F, *Land of Fish and Rice,* Bloomsbury Publishing, China, 2016.

Stoll, A L, *The Omega-3 Connection,* Simon & Schuster, 2001.

Stevenson, T, *Sotheby's World Wine Encyclopedia,* Dorling Kindersley, 1988

Weil, A, *Eating Well for Optimum Health,* Alfred Knopf, US, 2000.

Wilcox, B, J, Wilcox, D C, and Suzuki, M, *The Okinawa Program,* Three Rivers Press, New York, 2001.

Chapter eight

Cheung, J Y T, *Total Health and Fitness Revolution,* Possible Press, 2019.

Fontana, L, *The Path to Longevity,* Hardie Grant Books, London, 2020.

Liponis, M, *Ultra-Longevity,* Little Brown, 2007.

Sinclair, D, with LaPlante, M D, *Lifespan,* Thorson, London, 2019.

Your notes

Dr Joseph Cheung

Printed in Great Britain
by Amazon

10197313R00153